Intermittent Fasting
For Women 101

Eat What You Want, Take Care Of Your Body And
Health With This Proven Guide That Combines
The Effect On Fats Of The Keto Diet And The
Metabolic Autophagy Diet

Serena Weight

Legal & Disclaimer

The information contained in this book and its contents is not designed to replace or take the place of any form of medical or professional advice; and is not meant to replace the need for independent medical, financial, legal or other professional advice or services, as may be required. The content and information in this book has been provided for educational and entertainment purposes only.

The content and information contained in this book has been compiled from sources deemed reliable, and it is accurate to the best of the Author's knowledge, information and belief. However, the Author cannot guarantee its accuracy and validity and cannot be held liable for any errors and/or omissions. Further, changes are periodically made to this book as and when needed. Where appropriate and/or necessary, you must consult a professional (including but not limited to your doctor, attorney, financial advisor or such other professional advisor) before using any of the suggested remedies, techniques, or information in this book.

Upon using the contents and information contained in this book, you agree to hold harmless the Author from and against any damages, costs, and expenses, including any legal fees potentially resulting from the application of any of the information provided by this book. This disclaimer applies to any loss, damages or injury caused by the use and application, whether directly or indirectly, of any advice or information presented, whether for breach of contract, tort, negligence, personal injury, criminal intent, or under any other cause of action.

You agree to accept all risks of using the information presented inside this book.

You agree that by continuing to read this book, where appropriate and/or necessary, you shall consult a professional (including but not limited to your doctor, attorney, or financial advisor or such other advisor as needed) before using any of the suggested remedies, techniques, or information in this book.

Table of Contents

Introduction

Intermittent Fasting has been taking the health and fitness world by storm for decades. A practice as old as the human species and the survival instincts that helped develop us into the stable, healthy individuals of today. All over the world, people following all kinds of diets and all kinds of lifestyles are weaving fasting windows into their daily lives to help improve their physical and mental health and wellness progression. This guide has been specially created for women interested in Intermittent Fasting as a health and wellness tool to assist with reaching their personal health goals. The following chapters will cover not only the basics of Intermittent Fasting as a means of weight loss and health enhancement, but they will also cover topics that are specific to women health. By the end of the guide, readers will feel more comfortable with the concept of Intermittent Fasting and all that defines it so they can take their first steps with confidence and take advantage of all the benefits the program has to offer. Even though women need to take more exceptional care when preparing their Intermittent Fasting routines than men do, there is an abundance of positive health benefits women can gain from the right fasting schedule. Keep this book at your side throughout your Intermittent Fasting journey as a friend, a supporter, a guide and a quick reference when questions arise, or changes need to be made to your personal fasting schedule in order to maximize benefits or eliminate harmful side effects. There is no shortage of Intermittent Fasting books on the market and no limit of information available anywhere from social media to health and wellness community boards. Packed with useful and valuable information from cover to cover, Intermittent Fasting for Women is a robust planning and preparation tool for women interested in starting their first Intermittent Fasting plan. We hope you enjoy our guide and wish you every bit of luck on your personal health journey. The main goal of this guide is to be helpful in getting you to your best physical, mental, and emotional health with a strong and stable Intermittent Fasting routine personalized to help you meet your goals! This book is going to change your life! I know you just started reading, but I'm serious! My book is designed to impact your experience in the most positive way possible from a holistic standpoint. You probably decided to buy this book because you want to become a better version of yourself! You made the best investment to invest in your health and wellness. I got good news for you, and that is your life will be transformed once you start taking action and implementing these strategies I discuss within this book. Are you tired of being bombarded by countless infomercials that endorse new diet fads? I'm pretty sure you've heard it all from, ketogenic diet, paleo diet, vegan diet, and even the raw food diet. Now I'm not criticizing or taking jabs at any of these mentioned diets, and I do genuinely believe in most cases these diets do work effectively to a certain degree. But you see their lays an inherent problem with all these so-called "diets." People tend to go on them and start viewing some results, but before you know it, they start gaining back those unwanted pounds simply because they couldn't uphold their regiment. To add insult to injury, a lot of these diets tend to be more costly and run an expensive bill that cannot be sustained on the average working person's budget. Well, I'm here to tell you that intermittent Fasting won't cost you any more than you are already spending. This diet, in particular, is designed to help you burn unwanted body fat fast and sculpt your way to your ideal physique in conjunction to exercise. But, before we start discussing the basics, we need to get your mindset right! Something did not discuss a lot within the health and fitness industry, and that is having a good sense of self-awareness before you start any diet. You see the inherent problem I previously mentioned with all these diets is that people cannot uphold or continue on with certain diet regiments. Why? Because people treat diets like prescription drugs! Once results are derived, and an outcome is finalized, people tend to go back to their old ways of living and relegate their newfound diet fad to the back burner. You see, there is an inherent problem when you interface with a diet and consider it a short-term fix. Real transformation takes place from the inside out, and when you become aware of changing the way you eat is not a matter of going on a short term diet, but a total lifestyle change! That's right; you need to transform your lifestyle or modify it in order to achieve long-term sustainable results! You need to incorporate intermittent Fasting as apart of your daily living, and in order to do this, you need to shift your short term thinking to the long run. - This is not a prescription drug. Within the past few years, the concept of Intermittent Fasting has started to trend slowly, impacting anyone interested in dieting and healthy living. Its origins, however, are much more ancient than most of us would ever think. In this chapter, you'll be introduced to the long history of Intermittent Fasting so that you can better understand how that trajectory leads to today. By the end of this section, you should feel confident that you know where the tradition came from, as well as what it has to do with you—reading this book at this very moment.

Chapter 1: The History of Intermittent Fasting and contemporary applications

Fasting has been a natural part of life in one form or another since the origins of humankind. At its most basic level, fasting is a survival tool developed by early humans as a way to survive during long periods without food such as deep winter when many animals are in hibernation or after natural disasters such as plagues or floods when crops were unexpectedly destroyed. Instead of just giving into starvation or going straight to uprooting their community in search of more bountiful lands, they learned to restrict their calorie intake and ration their food to only consume enough to survive and make their reserves last until conditions improved.

Apart from survival, in countries and cultures across the planet, fasting is often most commonly associated with religious practice, devotion and ceremony. Long-standing religions with the most ancient roots are best known for this and incorporate a form of fasting into their beliefs.

Muslims of the Islamic belief fast during the holy month of Ramadan as a way of displaying their devotion to their beliefs for all to see. This form of fasting is more absolute than those used for medical and dieting purposes, eliminating even their water and liquid consumption during their 12-hour daily fasting windows (sunrise to sunset) and continuing their daily food consumption at night. Practitioners are free to eat normally within the dietary restrictions of Islam during eating windows and throughout the rest of the year.

- Due to the risk of serious digestive distress, potentially life-threatening dehydration and metabolic issues associated with increased calorie consumption during the evening hours just before bed, this form of fasting is not recommended for those using it as a means of improving their overall strength and wellness.

Christians are not required to fast for their religion but have used fasting for centuries as a means of getting closer to God. The practice is believed to prove an individual worshipper's true dedication, serve as a proper act of penance and strengthen their personal commitment through sacrifice and self-control. Forty days is the standard amount of time for experienced fasters, but some will fast on the holy day of Sunday while others will fast throughout the Catholic celebration of Lent.

Buddhism is another belief system famous for fasting as a form of devotion and discipline. Buddhism promotes a consistent form of Intermittent Fasting where people only eat in the early hours of the morning then start fasting at noon and continue to do so until the early hours of the next morning. The purpose of this is to practice self-discipline for the many physical and mental health benefits of fasting when practiced as a lifestyle and not just as a temporary health plan.

- This is another form of Intermittent Fasting that is not recommended by medical professionals and other health experts to be used as a means of weight loss as it can be difficult to adjust to, sometimes starting with an initial shock to the system that can increase fluid retention and fat storage in the body's cells.

Credit for the first use of fasting as a means of health improvement can be given to Hippocrates of Kos, a physician of ancient Greece most famous as the father of modern medicine and for being the inspiration for the Hippocratic oath. This oath is a pledge that new doctors take before they start their career promising to uphold high ethical standards and never cause any harm to another human being.

One of Hippocrates most commonly assigned treatments was to sip on apple cider vinegar in place of regular food consumption for a few days to a week, depending on the severity of the original illness or discomfort. The theory behind this was that the cause of the original sickness was something foul or tainted the patient consumed that affected he digestive tract and spread throughout the body from there. By not eating until the symptoms cleared, the patient's body was given the opportunity to heal without risk of consuming anything else toxic or fueling the sickness with calories and carbohydrates. The apple cider vinegar fought off starvation and kept the body functioning during the fasting period.

Intermittent Fasting Tip: Apple Cider Vinegar

Apple cider vinegar is still recommended today for detoxing and a number of other positive benefits such as:

- Apple cider vinegar, when regularly consumed, helps to balance pH levels in the body improving digestion, lowering blood sugar numbers and helps to boost energy.
- Apple cider vinegar has also been praised for its effectiveness in fighting cardiovascular disease and improving overall heart health.
- Apple cider vinegar is full of natural antioxidants that can help to fight basic illness such as the common cold and even help to strengthen the body's immune system to fight sickness year-round.
- **For Women:** Apple cider vinegar has a high level of calcium and has been proven to help with strengthening the body's bones and joints. This is one reason it is recommended for women who tend to have greater issues with skeletal degeneration over time than males do.

o Many doctors and dieticians recommend female patients consume one or two tablespoons of apple cider vinegar per day, diluted in water or undiluted depending on personal preference. Whether or not a woman decides to start fasting or go with a particular diet program, regular apple cider vinegar consumption for the purpose of increasing calcium levels is still a good habit to pick up.

Another theory for why the apple cider vinegar diet and fasting plan was (and is still) so effective is that avoiding food when feeling under the weather is a natural instinctive response anyway. This is one reason people tend to avoid heavy meals and gravitate towards hot tea and broth-based soups when they are not feeling well. This is another reason it works well when paired with lighter and liquid-based diets.

Why periodic fasting is not suitable for all women

The explanation is amazingly simple. As soon as the fetus is in the mother's stomach, it always secures its nutrients no matter what consequences this may have for the mother. The fetus is fighting for its survival. For this reason, pregnancy at the wrong time - e.g., during a hunger (= fasting) period can end badly for the mother.

Therefore, the stressors mentioned in some women can lead to unwant by effects. Scientists now believe that the energy balance is the main indicator of women's hormonal balance. With a negative energy balance, these hormonal changes can occur relatively quickly.

A negative energy balance often results from the following stressors:

• caloric deficit

• Unhealthy diet

• Too much stress

- Too long and intense training

- Diseases
- Not enough rest

What does all this mean exactly?

It means that IF is not suitable for all women. It does not mean that as a woman you must be scared now and not try IF. For most women, it works perfectly well. It just means that you have to be a little more careful and listen to your body.

For who is intermittent fasting NOT suitable?
In the following cases, IF is probably not for you, or you should stop trying:

- Your period is suspended

- You have sleep problems

- You are in a state of anxiety

- Your recovery after training worsens

- Hair fall out

- Your body feels colder than normal

- Your mood is getting worse

- Your skin is irritated

- You have less desire for sex

Before you panic ... 99% of women probably will not.

But the fact is that IF should not be an issue for some women:

- Pregnant women because they need more energy

- Chronically stressed women, because for them IF is just another stressor

- Women with insomnia, because only these need to be treated

The best tip is to listen to your body. You'll soon realize if is right for you (and that does not mean you should give up after 1-2 days just because you're hungry during fasting, which is normal as long as your body is not used to it), Intermittent fasting is an excellent strategy to lose weight quickly and painlessly and to live longer at the same time.

But the fact is that IF is not suitable for everyone. Especially women who are under a lot of stress should keep their hands off it. And of course, it must be said that it varies from person to person. For most, it works perfectly well and for some not at all. You just have to try it yourself. That's the best tip for you.

Chapter 2 – Benefits of intermittent fasting

Now that the basics of Intermittent Fasting as a health enhancement option have been laid out, this guide is going to cover the specifics of Intermittent Fasting as it relates to women and their personal health. As women who have been working out or dieting throughout the course of their lives know, not every program that guarantees progress for men will work for females following the same steps, routine or health menu.

In this chapter, we'll take a look at some of the differences in Intermittent Fasting between male and female participants, introduce the first of our simple steps to mastering Intermittent fasting for women, and provide some helpful tips and tricks to getting started on your own Intermittent Fasting journey!

Intermittent Fasting & The Female Form

There are a number of factors from the biological to the hormonal that can affect the success of a dieting, nutrition or fitness program for women. Some of the negative risks and effects that women see more than men do when starting a new Intermittent Fasting routine include:

- **Hormonal imbalance-** Hormonal imbalances in women can evolve into a wide variety of more serious concerns related to biology and genetics. Some of these concerns include irregular menstruation (length of period or strength of flow) or changes in skin tone and sudden, difficult to clear blemishes.
- **Excessive fatigue-** Fatigue and muscle weakness are two common side effects that come with severely cutting calorie intake, but these are increased for women as the female body relies more on glucose and fat storage to

function. While over time the negative side effects decrease or even disappear, the initial transition and adapting to a fasting schedule (depending also on how intense the fasting plan is) is typically more difficult in the first few weeks.

- **Emotional instability-** Also often related to fluctuating hormones, mood swings are a common problem reported by women following an Intermittent Fasting plan, especially in the first two weeks to one month.

It's not all health concerns and difficulties! There are lots of ways that women can benefit from adding an Intermittent Fasting schedule into their daily routine and developing it into their lifestyle in order to help enhance their overall health.

How Does Intermittent Fasting Benefit Women?

Intermittent Fasting is one way that has been shown to assist women with high cholesterol levels, existing heart conditions or heavy risk of heart disease with working on improving their numbers and health options (along with the help of a personal physician or medical professional). This is just one of many health benefits women who have adopted Intermittent Fasting into their daily lifestyle have reported and praised.

Other widely reported positive health effects include:

- Lower risk for the development of and effective treatment of chronic diseases
- Reduced risk of and assistance with controlling obesity
- Women have shown more positive results in the treatment of Type 2 Diabetes and other blood sugar-related conditions with Intermittent Fasting thanks to the increased insulin production the body experiences

- Reduced inflammation throughout the body for those with chronic diseases, lower blood pressure and greater control over blood pressure-related conditions
- Intermittent Fasting has proven to be one of the most effective ways for women having trouble getting rid of stubborn fat deposits to finally burn them off, particularly in places like the core and thighs

Women going through menopause have reported Intermittent Fasting as playing a major role in their losing extra weight gained with their hormonal fluctuations. Others have reported seeing more positive stability in their emotional states and the ability to control their emotional impulses throughout the day. The full effects are still being studied on human participants, but in the last decade, tests featuring the effects of Intermittent Fasting on female rats in their menopausal stage have shown encouraging results leading to Intermittent Fasting being more widely recommended for women who are struggling with controlling their menopause symptoms.

While the health benefits of Intermittent Fasting for women specifically are promising, they are still being studied and it is important to remember that everyone's experience with fasting will be different thanks to the personal health factors, biological factors, lifestyle and diet factors, along with any other number of variables that can affect the effectiveness of fasting for individuals.

How Is Intermittent Fasting Riskier for Women?

Female participants in studies across the globe and those reporting their personal results on social media or within fitness communities report many of the same negative effects felt by men throughout the course of adjusting to a new Intermittent Fasting plan. Some of these side effects include:

- Initial hunger pangs and dehydration

- Difficulty concentrating or gaining focus throughout the day
- Headaches, muscle weakness, initial loss in muscle tone

There are some effects that women have experienced and should be watched out for, especially those with a history of trouble or concerns with their menstrual cycles. One such negative effect reported is infertility after long periods of time on an Intermittent Fasting plan. This tends to happen more in women who see a dramatic loss in body fat, especially in the first few weeks (or during the adjustment time).

- In most women, this is nothing to be permanently concerned about as typically periods return to normal and fertility increases in the weeks after stopping an Intermittent Fasting plan, particularly for weight loss reasons
- Most wellness experts and medical professionals recommend that women who may be pregnant, are pregnant or are hoping to become pregnant in the near future avoid starting or cease their Intermittent Fasting plan in order to ensure they are in peak condition for childbearing or do not minimize their chances of conceiving

However, for those worried about starting an Intermittent Fasting routine, it is important to point out that even though fasting is still being studied around the world for its long-term benefits and risks on nearly anyone who could ever be interested in trying it (different ages, genders, races, cultural diets, health histories), health and wellness experts all over have written and spoken about its safety, its benefits and its promising progress for men and women alike. It all comes down to being prepared; having all the right information and making a plan that will work and can be stuck with for the long run.

Types of intermittent Fasting

The very first thing you have to know about intermittent fasting is that it is not a diet! It can be viewed as a lifestyle choice that you make to eliminate a few meals and snacks per day. But do not confuse it with starvation, as you have to eat to provide your body with enough energy and nutrients to keep you going.

The intermittent fast is a simple concept where you alternate between periods of eating and fasting. It is a matter of knowing when to eat as opposed to what to eat. It calls for the consumption of everyday calories within a certain period of time and remaining in fasting phase for the rest of the day.

Here are some of the fasting plans to choose from.

The 16/8 fast

The 16/8 diets is one version where you fast for 16 hours and eat in the next 8 hours. It is a very simple plan. All you have to do is figure out a period when you would like to consume your normal three meals. Say, for example, you have your dinner by 8 p.m. The next meal has to be consumed only after 12 noon the next day. You will have to skip breakfast and go for lunch instead. It is your choice to have 3 meals or limit it to two, i.e., lunch, snack and dinner or lunch and dinner in the next 8 hours.

This intermittent fast is easier to adopt for those who are accustomed to skipping breakfast. All you have to do is ensure you do not consume anything in the fasting hours. You are, however, allowed to have liquids. You can have any type of liquid including juices; fruit infused water, coconut water, etc. Just make sure you keep a tab on the calorie level and avoid sugary drinks or those with calories.

The 5:2 fast

The 5:2 intermittent fast is a version that is designed to help you shed excess weight within a few months. It is one where you consume a regular diet for 5 days and fast on the remaining 2 days. These 2 days can be weekends or any two days of your choice. It is not advisable to go completely without food on these two days. Limit your calorie intake to 500 or 600. There are no restrictions as to what you can have for the remaining 5 days. Men should limit it to 600 and women should go for 500 calories on the fasting days.

Warrior diet

The warrior diet is a rather simple form of intermittent fast. It can be considered as a beginner's intermittent fast. All you have to do is go for small portions of vegetables and fruit in the mornings. You then have a regular meal at night. There is no restriction on what you can consume for dinner. The warrior diet is so called because athletes and sportsmen trying to get fit follow this plan.

Eat stop eat

The eat stop eat is a type of diet that is said to be on the extreme side. It calls for you to not eat anything for an entire day. This is only ideal if you are accustomed to fasting. If you are not, then you might end up sending your body into starvation mode. So, ensure that you only take up this diet if you are comfortable with the idea of not consuming a meal for 24 hours straight. Let's say you consume your meal at 2 p.m. The next has to be consumed at 2 p.m. the next day. There are no restrictions to what can be consumed the rest of the week.

Alternate fasting

This is an extension of the previous type of fast where you fast on alternate days. If you eat your regular three meals on Sunday then you fast on Monday, eat again on Tuesday and fast on Wednesday and so on. Keep alternating between fasting and eating. This can be quite taxing and should be followed by those who are prepared for it. You can always consume liquids on fasting days. They have to be controlled in terms of calorie intake. It is best to go for this diet during the last few stages of weight loss. Start with the 16/8 and then go for the 5:2 before going for the eat stop eat version and then gradually take on alternate fasting.

The choice is yours. Choose any of these fasting types to get started with intermittent fasting. Here are some tips to help you.

• Make sure you choose the correct time frame to have your meals and stick to it. The idea behind the intermittent fast is that you try and reduce the number of meals you consume per day. Most of us are accustomed to consuming three meals a day with 2 or 3 snacks thrown in between. The intermittent fast aims at reducing the number of meals consumed to 2 meals per day.

• The idea is to go from an 8-hour eating window to 6-hour window and finally to a 4-hour window.

• The best way to go about this is by first taking on the 8-hour eating window and cutting out the morning snack. This snack is usually consumed between breakfast and lunch. Most of us start feeling puckish at around the 12-noon mark and reach for something to munch on. Having this snack cannot only make you delay your lunch; it can also make you go back on your fast. So, a good idea would be to consume a heavy breakfast. Eat at least 450 calories and include an egg omelet with an avocado shake. For lunch, go for 450 calories and have chicken curry with flatbread. For dinner, go for something light such as a vegetable salad and a glass of fresh juice.

• The next challenge would be to cut out the evening snack. According to research, those who consume a late evening or late-night snack end up gaining weight much more easily. Make sure you do not dig into a snack before dinner. Start your day with the same menu as mentioned in the previous point. Consume a heavier lunch of about 500 calories. Keep dinner simple and limit it to 400 calories.

• By following the previous two steps, you will have successfully gone from 5 meals a day to 3 by cutting out two snacks. The next step would be to cut out one of the meals.

• It might sound like you are being asked not to eat anything at all. But it is not the case as you can pack in the same number of calories within two meals. The meal you wish to drop depends on you. Some prefer to do away with breakfast while some prefer to skip lunch and others forgo dinner. Since you know your body best, it is entirely up to you to choose which two meals to go for.

• Once you have decided on the meals, the next step is to start narrowing down the eating window. If you are used to eating at 12 noons followed by lunch at 4 p.m. and dinner by 8 p.m., then eliminate lunch and go for heavier breakfast and dinner.

• Next, close the gap between the two by having lunch at 1 p.m. and dinner at 7 p.m. This will bring down the eating window to 6 hours. Continue this for a couple of weeks.

• Next, reduce the eating window to 4-hours. Have your lunch by 2 p.m. and your dinner by 6 p.m. This can sound a bit daunting but taking it up can help you build a strong and healthy body. In fact, it can alter your thought process and make you a productive and happy person.

• Remember to have visual reminders everywhere. Paste your meal plan on the fridge door so that you are motivated to stick to it.

• Bear in mind that not all calories are the same. You have to know what to eat and what to avoid. Just because you are eating just two meals doesn't mean you go for junk and processed foods. These should never be an option. The calories should come by way of healthy foods. Don't worry about cutting down on a majority of the meals. You are not denying your body anything. You are only modifying the structure of meal consumption.

•   Apart from meal consumption, you must also focus on sleeping well. The more you sleep, the more calories your body burns. When you sleep, your body automatically starts burning calories. If there are fewer calories to burn, then it will start drawing from your fat reserves. This means that you do not even have to exercise and that sleep alone will do the job for you.

•   It is also very easy for you to take on the diet if you push your fasting periods to night times. When you sleep, you are less likely to crave food. You will also not feel like getting up and grabbing something to eat. This will make it easier for you to stick to the fast.

•   Remember that it is always best to eat your last meal as early as possible. Think of consuming it by 5 p.m. if possible and sleep by 9 p.m. This will catapult your weight loss process.

Chapter 3: The effects on fats of ketogenic diet and metabolic diet

Weight loss is one of the most important reasons why people implement an intermittent fasting program in their lives. The weight loss benefits of this eating plan have been proven – in addition to assisting with metabolism, the diet also helps to curb your appetite, which means you will eat less.

With intermittent fasting, it is essential that you understand it is possible to gain weight instead of to lose weight if your diet is not appropriate. You will need to implement an appropriate diet in order to ensure that you achieve a caloric deficit, while still providing your body with the essential nutrients it relies on daily to perform all of the functions that are crucial to your own survival.

Different types of meal plans have been suggested for those people who are looking to lose weight through intermittent fasting. In the end, it is up to you to choose a meal plan that is appropriate for you. You will have to take yourself into account – consider how much weight you have to lose, and take into account any particular health conditions that you may be suffering from.

The first step to losing weight with this type of eating habit would be to select an appropriate type of intermittent fasting program. We have already discussed the various options out there that you can select from. Most people find that the standard 16/8 intermittent fasting program is ideal for them if they are only getting started. You can vary the number of days during the week that you will be following this program – some are also able to follow through with the 16/8 program for the entire week. You'll essentially have to listen to your own body – when you feel that you are starving yourself too much, adjust your plan in order to make up for the excessive reduction in your daily caloric consumption. On the other hand, if you find that you are not losing weight, it might be a good idea to take a look at your calorie balance – how much calories are you consuming and how much are you burning through physical activity?

Autophagy ranks high among the most popular methods of weight management and healthy living, and this process is termed autophagy for a reason. Most people who have tried it can relate the benefits they have derived and the ways it has improved their life. But then, what is autophagy?

Do you suffer from recurrent body pains? Are you easily prone to illness, or do you find it difficult to shed some weight? Then, all you need to do is to acquire more knowledge of autophagy and the fasting processed involved.

This book will enlighten you on what autophagy is all about, the benefits associated with it and many more.

- Here is a clue of what lies ahead:
- All about autophagy; how it works, how to induce it, and its benefits
- Benefits and side effects of fasting, and precautions to take when fasting
- How to ease into fasting, doing it the right and easy way, and understanding your routine

Everyone needs autophagy in their lives, and no one benefits from being overweight; rather, being overweight poses some health risks. Being overweight can cause inflammation, heart-related diseases as well as others.

Can you imagine how active and alive you will feel after losing some weight within a few weeks into autophagy? Furthermore, imagine how happy your friends and family will be when they see you radiating with more energy than ever before? All these benefits can be achieved with less stress and without starving yourself to death.

Over time, the metabolic activities in a healthy human body lead to cellular damage. Sadly, the rate at which our cells are damaged increases as we age due to stress, exposure to radiation among others. However, Autophagy can help the body remove such damaged cells as well as old cells that are no longer active but are still present in the body. If such cells are not removed, it may lead to inflammatory diseases as well as other harmful cardiovascular diseases.

Autophagy is derived from the combination of two Greek words, which are: auto, which means 'self', and phage, which means to 'engulf.' Therefore, autophagy means the engulfment of the body's cells or tissues as part of the normal metabolic processes, which is both beneficial and protective.

Over the years, fasting has been used as a way of shedding weight.

The Origin of Autophagy

Early in the 1950s, Christian de Duve a Belgian scientist discovered the process of autophagy by accident while working on insulin.

Between 1970 and 1980, researchers began taking a closer look at the process of cellular autophagy. At that time, little information was available about the importance of autophagy. After so many years of hard work, a significant milestone was achieved in 1983, when Yoshinori Osama, discovered genes responsible for the regulation of autophagy in yeast. From his discovery, he found out that autophagy was absent in yeast cells lacking those genes and such cells were unable to repair themselves. In 2016, he was awarded a Nobel Prize for this great discovery.

The interesting thing about this discovery is how the cell responds to increased stress, nutrient deficiency, deprivation of energy and cellular injuries by increasing the rate of cellular autophagy but where the stress is eliminated, the process of autophagy goes back to the regular rate (maintenance mode).

With more desires to fully understand the process of autophagy, more research works are now aimed at understanding the relationship between aging and autophagy, and the effect of stress on this process.

There is a general theory that there is a relationship between aging and the rate of autophagy as well. According to evidence, the process that enhances autophagy will also help to extend the lifespan of such individual. Another research reported that cell related aging attributed to the accumulation of damaged cells without proper means of removal. Since autophagy helps to remove damaged cells thereby slowing down the process of aging, scientists are looking at ways of extending the life expectancy of humans by inducing autophagy.

Chapter 4: The science of intermittent Fasting

The human body has two main settings that determine how efficient, powerfully and smoothly our internal systems run. They help to boost energy throughout the day and provide extra fuel from stored fat cells to injured areas to help speed the healing process.

#1 Store Fat for Later Use: When people consume carbohydrates, sugars, and excess protein, the body digests it and uses it for the energy and nutrition it needs now, then transfers the remainder to the liver where it is converted into glycogen to be stored in fat deposits around the body in case of emergency. This is the process most active in the human body during feeding or feasting windows when food is being consumed regularly. When humans eat, the insulin production levels of the body increase thanks to the consumed sugars being digested and deposited in the liver as fat cells. When the liver itself can't hold any more fat but the human continues to eat, all new fat created from ingested food travels to other storage areas such as the core and thighs.

#2 Burn Stored Fat for Extra Fuel: This process is the one most active in times of fasting. Instead of relying on glucose delivered from food sources, the body is able to call upon stored fat cells to convert into emergency energy for the internal organs or body processes. This is the body's natural survival defense against starvation and can happen in times of distress such as being lost or at the mercy of harsh weather. It is also a process that can be initiated and controlled without risk of fatality or illness with Intermittent Fasting. It is monitored and upheld by a person's fluctuating glucose levels. When this begins, the body switches from running on empty sugar cells to burning excess fat so it can maintain energy until individual eats again.

Intermittent Fasting works by creating (and sticking to) a fasting schedule designed to control when the body slips in and out of these processes to minimize fat storage and maximize fat burning.

Intermittent Fasting For Cancer Prevention

Intermittent fasting reduces the development and progression of tumors in animal experiments. Rats on IF transplanted with a cancer cell line survived longer than free-fed animals. After 10 days, 50% of the IF animals were still alive compared to 12.5% in the control group.

Alternating fasting used only in middle age reduced the incidence of lymphoma in mice. In a 4-month observation period, 30% of the control mice became ill while none of the animals on intermittent fasting became cancerous. The researchers also found a better antioxidant activity, resulting in less development of harmful free radicals within the mitochondria (cell power plants). The antitumor effect did not result from the calorie reduction since both groups consumed the same amount of calories.

In rats, intermittent fasting reduced the development of pre-neoplastic (precursor to cancer) liver injury and liver nodules caused by a carcinogenic substance.

Unfortunately, human studies do not exist so far.

Lowered Cardiovascular Risk

In one study, intermittent fasting in non-obese participants resulted in an increase in good HDL cholesterol in women and a reduction in triglyceride levels in men. This effect occurred over 22 days in which every two days fasted. This change may have been caused by the degradation of body fat, which was -4%.

In the case of obese people, the values improved more clearly by an average weight loss of -5.6 kg after eight weeks of alternating fasting.

Total cholesterol dropped by 21%, LDL cholesterol by 25% and triglycerides by 32% while HDL cholesterol remained unchanged.

The systolic blood pressure dropped from 124 to 116 mmHg.

Stress resistance induced by intermittent fasting has a cardio protective effect beyond reducing body weight. Studies in mice show that in a heart attack, the affected tissue in the heart is half-smaller in alternately fasting mice than in normally fed animals. Also, in cardiac infarction, 4 times fewer cardiocytes die (heart muscle cells), when the animals were fed intermittently.

Calorie Independent Effect

Calorie restriction can have a positive effect on health and life expectancy. Some intermittent fasting researchers and advocates claim that starvation is more important than actually reducing calorie intake. Because fasting is a kind of stress for the body, it could stimulate the expression of genes that perform protective tasks and theoretically bring health benefits.

Some nutritionists assume that our ancestors did not consistently have food supplies, but were instead exposed to hunger periods and periods of increased caloric intake and those there genes were shaped and adapted accordingly. Thus, an alternate availability of food would be "natural."

IF partially dissociates the positive effect of calorie reduction from the actual total intake of calories. In mice, intermittent fasting results in improved glucose control, lower insulin levels, and greater resistance to neuronal damage regardless of weight loss or calorie intake.

Even without a reduction in calories, intermittent fasting increases the concentration of the hormone adiponectin. Adiponectin increases fat burning, anti-inflammatory, and antidiabetic and has a positive influence on cardiovascular health.

Distribution of fat deposits

In mice, intermittent fasting even without a weight loss leads to a redistribution of fat deposits in the body. The fat shifts from the visceral (in the abdomen) to the subcutaneous (under the skin) body fat. This change is healthier because visceral body fat is associated with increased inflammatory levels, insulin resistance, and metabolic syndrome. Although advocates often mention this effect of intermittent fasting, clinical studies have so far failed to detect a particularly increased decrease in visceral adipose tissue in humans.

Unfortunately, most versions of intermittent fasting, such as Eat Stop Eat, do not give users a healthy dietary change. The existing eating habits and the choice of food to be maintained, the method should only be a simplification to facilitate the calorie abstinence, however, a relearning is not promoted, which makes it easy to relapse into old habits, especially in obese people. There is a risk of migration between extremes: on the one hand fasting and on the other hand food cravings paired with the choice of low-nutrient and low-fiber, but high-calorie diet.

On the other hand, intermittent fasting provides a straightforward way to lose weight and, like any other diet, works better in some people than in others, depending on preference.

Fasting over 24 hours due to calorie restriction in calorie intake overshadows the negative effects on circadian rhythms caused by intermittent fasting, which merely shifts the meal timeslots towards evening (especially warrior diet, lean gains in part).

Side Effects

Intermittent fasting is usually very well tolerated, for some users the first few days on which they starve for longer are unusual and can cause irritation, fatigue or euphoria.

A double-blind, placebo-controlled, two-day study in which participants did not know if they were receiving any caloric or calorie-free food (in gel form) could not identify any side effects related to mental performance, physical activity, sleep, and whim.

A 24-hour Lent, without excessive exercise, lowers glycogen storage in the liver by almost 60%, so that the stored carbohydrates can easily maintain the blood sugar at a sufficient level. After 24 hours of fasting, the blood sugar level does not reach a pathological level (hypoglycemia). Also, the body can at any time through the process of gluconeogenesis produce sugar from amino acids and rely on ketones as a source of energy for the nervous system. However, this is unlikely as muscle breakdown in intermittent fasting is lower than in other diets, suggesting a muscle-sparing effect.

Diabetes 2 Risk

Humane studies have so far only observed a positive change in diabetes 2-related factors in men. Intermittent fasting increased insulin-mediated glucose uptake after 2 weeks, suggesting improved insulin sensitivity. These results are supported by another study in which male participants release less insulin after a 3-week alternating fast (always 36-hour fasting) in response to a meal, another indication of increased insulin sensitivity and thus a reduction in the risk of diabetes 2 Intermittent fasting, Women, on the other hand, developed inferior glucose tolerance during the same treatment because they had elevated blood sugar levels after a test meal.

At this point, it is essential to consider the small number of participants in the respective studies who can by no means provide definitive answers.

Aging Process

The restriction of calorie intake (calorie restriction, CR) is one of the most reliable methods to increase the lifespan of animals in animal studies significantly. Calorie restriction generally means a 10-30% daily reduction in daily caloric intake, resulting in an increase in the life span of various organisms from yeast, worms to nonhuman primates.

Calorie restriction is associated with improved insulin sensitivity, lowering of heart rate and blood pressure (which benefits cardiovascular health), reduced free radical damage to cellular components (proteins, DNA), reduced incidence of spontaneous and induced tumors and better resistance of neurons degenerative changes.

Intermittent fasting is an alternative to daily calorie restriction, with a similar effect on the aging process and lifespan. Alternating fasting in mice resulted in an extension of the average lifespan by 2.8-6.7 months when fasting was introduced at a young age. Several theories try to explain life-prolonging and health effects. Among other things, the stress caused by the calorie withdrawal could cause an overreaction of defense mechanisms, which allow the cells better defense against metabolic, genotoxic and oxidative stress, Intermittent fasting may be similar in effect to caloric restriction, but may be different, as the stress caused by starvation is more intense.

Brain Power and Aging

Both calorie restriction and intermittent fasting affect neuronal functionality, which decreases with age.

With advancing age, the so-called spine processes, which are located at the dendrites (branched cell processes) of neurons (nerve cells), decrease. The spine processes play an important role in the information transfer between the nerve cells. In rats, the number of thorns decreased by 38% after 24 months of a normal diet.

Intermittent fasting prevented the reduction of the density of the spine so that rats showed little difference to 6-month-old rats even after 24 months.

Calorie reduction by the intermittent fasting increased neurogenesis (formation of new brain cells), protected the neurons from dying and stimulated the production of BDNF (brain-derived neurotrophic factor), a protein associated with increased neurogenesis, in this way, if counteracts the deterioration of the aging process and improves the learning ability of older mice.

The effect on neurogenesis also appears to promote healing and functional recovery of spinal cord injuries in animals, whether intermittent fasting was introduced before or shortly after injury.

Chapter 5: Understanding and Functions of autophagy

Autophagy, when broken down, translates from Greek to mean "self-eating." This is a normal, biological process in the human body that occurs on the cellular level, deep within the cytoplasm. Breaking down the cell and its components can shed more light on why autophagy occurs in the first place.

The basic cell of any human is made of proteins, lipids, cholesterol, and water, and these components make up the mechanisms that encourage healthy cell performance.

A cell is a sophisticated machine comprised of many organelles, plasma, amino acids, glucose, genetic information, and chemical compounds that help the cell to perform its functions. Here is a breakdown of what you will find within every cell in the body, no matter what body system it is working in:

Nucleus

The nucleus has a double membrane and is a spherical shape containing your DNA strands. This part of the cells dictates protein synthesis, playing a major role in our cell performance, most specifically active transport of genetic information, metabolism, growth, and heredity.

Nucleoli

A dense region, and part of the nucleus, the nucleoli play a major part in the creation of ribosomes.

Ribosome

Tiny particles in the cell made of rRNA sub-particles. The job of the ribosome is to synthesize proteins. It is often referred to as the protein factory of the cell.

Cilia

These are short, hair-like extensions on the outer surface of the cell that can move substances or particles over the outer surface.

Plasma Membrane

This is the phospholipid layer of the skin of the cell. It is studded with proteins and serves as the cell's gatekeeper, the castle wall. When there are carbohydrates and proteins on the outer side of the cell, they will perform certain functions connected to the plasma membrane such as allowing for individual cell identification as a receptor for certain hormones, like the gatekeepers at the gate.

Mitochondria

This organelle is a network of membranous folds covered in enzymes and is where your ATP, or adenosine triphosphate, is synthesized. They are referred to as the cell powerhouses, creating energy on the microscopic level for the whole body.

Lysosomes

A round, bubble-like organelle, covered in a membrane, the lysosome is the digestive system or recycling center of the cell.

Centrioles

A pair of hollow cylinders made up of tiny tubules, the function of the centriole is cell reproduction.

Golgi Apparatus

A stack of flat, membranous sacs, the Golgi apparatus chemically processes and packages substances from the endoplasmic reticulum.

Endoplasmic Reticulum (ER)

There is rough ER and smooth ER. Rough ER is covered in ribosomes, while smooth ER has no attached organelles. The ER is a network of sacs and canals and has a membranous quality.

Every human cell performs certain functions. Some functions of the cell are to maintain its own survival, and other functions are to maintain the body's survival. Most of the time, the number and type of organelles allow the cells to differ dramatically regarding how they specifically function. For example, cells that contain a large number of mitochondria, such as cardiovascular muscle cells, are capable of sustained work. The excess of mitochondria can synthesize more ATP to have more energy in the cell; they can support the necessary energy required for ongoing rhythmic contractions. Movement of the flagellum of sperm, the only cell in the body to have a flagellum (tail), is another example of a specialized organelle and its specific function. The sperm, a cell in the male reproductive system, is propelled by the flagellum through the reproductive tract of the female, increasing the chances of fertilization. Every cell has a distinct purpose and health.

All cells require some movement bringing things in and pushing things out. The movement of substances through cells is a major aspect of our ability to live healthfully. If our cells reject nutrient because they are unable to absorb any, then you and your cells will suffer.

The plasma membrane in a healthy cell separates the contents of the cell from the tissue fluid that surrounds it. At the same time, the membrane has to permit certain substances and chemical compounds to enter the cell and allow others to depart. Heavy traffic moves continuously in both directions through all cell membranes. Things like water molecules, food molecules, gases, wastes, and many others flow in and out of cells in an endless procession. There are two general ways this process occurs: **passive** and **active** transport processes.

Active transport requires the expenditure of energy by the cell; passive transport does not. The energy required for the active transport process is obtained through ATP or adenosine triphosphate. ATP is created in the mitochondria of the cell, using energy from nutrients, and is capable of releasing that energy to do work within the cell. For active transport to occur, the breakdown of ATP and use of that released energy are required.

The details of active and passive transport are much easier to understand if you remember two key facts:

1. Passive transport—no cellular energy is required to move substances from a high to a low concentration.

2. Active transport—cellular energy is required to move substances from a low to a high concentration.

Within each kind of transport, you can break it down further to understand the function of the cell and how it operates to stay healthy and perform the various functions that work to keep the body alive. For example, within passive transport processes, there is diffusion, which includes osmosis and dialysis and filtration; within active transport processes, there is the ion pump, phagocytosis, and pinocytosis.

Active transport processes are what autophagy explains. Phagocytosis is most closely linked to the concept of autophagy. Autophagy is similar in that is the eating of materials within the cell. And like the transport processes, autophagy has its own variations that you will read about in the next chapter.

Bringing these concepts into a frame, consider the process of autophagy from the perspective of the lysosome.

The **lysosome** is the part of the cell to pay particular attention to when learning and understanding autophagy. It has the nickname "digestive bags" in some biological documents because of its particular job within the cell. They contain the enzymes that digest food substances. It isn't just food that they digest; they are also responsible for the digestion of microbes that invade the cell, and waste materials collected in the cell that need to be removed. Lysosomes protect the cell against destruction; they are also, in a way, the immune system of the cell.

The lysosome searches for pieces and parts of old, worn down, and discarded cell material, such as dead organelles, damaged proteins, oxidized particles, and other bio-waste. The cells absorb the waste matter and collect useful components to build new cell parts. It is essentially your body's recycling system that occurs on a microscopic level. This process is what allows the body to eliminate faulty, errant organisms, a cancerous growth, and cell metabolism dysfunction.

Autophagy is not to be confused with apoptosis, which is the death of the entire cell. Apoptosis is normal and occurs as a part of cell growth and development. Autophagy is the removal of dead or dysfunctional bio-matter in the cell, some of which is recycled and repaired for future use, rather than overall death of the whole machine. It is the body's system for cleaning house. Unlike our own digestive system, our cells cannot simply flush their waste down the toilet.

This process is also known to assist in your body's ability to have strong immunity and fight inflammation, which can lead to a variety of health issues. Some inflammation is beneficial to your body, as when you are fighting a cold or healing from an acute wound, however, regular existence of inflammation in your body can break down your cellular function and lead to dysfunction. When you break it down, autophagy is our body's way of keeping us healthy, cancer-free, fit, energized, mentally well, and living longer. It is an adaptive response in the face of all stress.

When cells are stressed, such as lacking nutrients, energy, insulin, or become damaged from chronic variations of all of the above, a stress response occurs which initiates autophagy.

What is healthy stress? Exercise, fasting, and ketosis. Without this kind of healthy stress, our cells will perform moderately and not optimally, suggesting that if you want to induce a serious, healing change in your body, you need to induce autophagy with the appropriate stress.

Autophagy is considered beneficial for many reasons, including the rejuvenation of the cells to impact life-long health and balance. When your cells age the machinery within, the cell also ages and becomes dysfunctional or nonfunctional. Autophagy is a biological maneuver to refresh and renew the cell by eliminating waste or recycling it for more efficient use and performance. By this method of cellular repair, the idea is that you can activate autophagy intentionally to promote cell rejuvenation that will reduce chances of certain age-related illnesses, diseases, and disorders. It can also repair existing conditions like diabetes, obesity, and food and health-related disorders that are the result of poor diet and lack of exercise. Several studies have shown improvement in neurodegenerative disorders, too, such as Parkinson's and Alzheimer's.

Think of it like the cell-cleansing garbage disposal crew. We have our own self-cleaning system when our cells are dirty with a build-up of old waste. It can represent in the way we feel and even the way we look. If you have dry, flaky skin and limp damaged hair, it may be due to the cell clutter that hasn't been able to clean for some reason. If you are fatigued, overweight, and aching all over, it may be because your cells cannot perform optimally under those conditions. Looking deeper into the cell will tell you more about the functions of autophagy.

Benefits of Fasting:

1. It enhances the body's fitness. Fasting helps the body to burn fats, and as such, the body will feel lighter and such individual can be said to be fit.

2. Promotes greater satiety. Your adipocytes produce various hormones (acting as an endocrine organ), such as your leptin, which regulates the way you feel. When you fast; however, you burn most of these stored fatty tissues, your leptin levels drop automatically (creating a leptin-deficient environment). Hence, whenever the little amount of leptin is produced, the effect is heightened, and your body becomes more responsive to leptin thereby modulating how you feel after a meal.

3. Enhanced metabolism. Leptin is also known as the (satiety hormone) also stimulate the production of thyroid hormones. Thus, enhanced leptin responsiveness will directly increase the rate of metabolism.

4. Facilitates fat loss and ketosis. Fat-loss or ketosis can be accomplished either by eating a Ketogenic Diet or by fasting. A Ketogenic Diet helps to burn out stored fat, which is harmful rather than helpful to the body organs such as the liver, the kidneys, and the blood vessels.

5. Enhances insulin sensitivity: When you fast, the body secretes a lesser amount of insulin, which in turn increases insulin sensitivity.

6. Boosts cardiovascular health: Fasting is recommended for those who wish to improve their cardiovascular function and have normal blood pressure.

7. Reduced blood pressure. Most people experience lower BP while fasting. This effect could be as a result of lower salt consumption and increased salt loss through urine.

8. Lower blood sugar. The blood sugar could drop as much as over 30 percent within a few days of fasting, and if care is not taken, the person could become hyperglycemic.

9. Decreases blood triglycerides. The triglycerides content of the blood drops low while an individual is fasting which helps to increase the blood flow within the blood vessels, which could have been narrowed by fat components.

10. Better heart condition. Fasting has been found to help reduce the accumulation of free radicals within the body. Free radicals are harmful to the muscles of the heart.

11. Could slow the rate of aging and prolong your lifespan. There have been positive results obtained from animal studies to prove that fasting could prolong lifespan. Also, when the blood is cleaned regularly, it slows down the process of aging and improves the health of an individual.

12. Suppresses inflammation. Although several factors cause inflammation, an unhealthy diet could lead to increased production of free radicals, which in turn could cause inflammation. Food items such as alcohol, refined food items, fried foods, etc. are all sources of free radicals.

13. Reduces the effects of Oxidative Stress. When the rate at which free radicals are produced is higher than the rate at which it is eliminated, it accumulates in the body thereby causing oxidative stress, which is damaging to the cells of the body.

14. Enhances cellular recycling process. Senescent cells accumulate in our body as we age. But when we fast, the body activates the process of self-digestion, and along the line, malignant cells are also destroyed.

15. Growth regulation. It has been found that insulin-like growth factor 1 (IGF-1) could lead to the proliferation of cancer. But fasting suppresses the production of IGF-1.

16. Protects the brain. Research works carried out on the function of the brain and aging has revealed one could age gracefully by fasting regularly.

17. Promotes a healthy stress response. Moderate stress is beneficial to the brain especially when it is infrequent, and fasting can induce such stress. Moderate stress triggers a series of activities that are protective to the brain cells (neurons).

18. Promotes recovery from an injury. Though the mechanism is not fully understood, research from animal models has shown that intermittent fasting helps the healing process.

19. Supports healthier skin collagen production. Your skin is a reflection of your diet. Accumulation of glucose can compromise the structure of the collagen, but fasting can help you overcome this challenge and give your skin that glow.

Side Effects of Fasting

Everyone fasts for various reasons such as: to lose weight, for a religious purpose, for healthy living and the list go on. A fast could either be mild or strict (ranging from liquid only such as juice, tea, coffee and the likes to no food, no fluid). Although fasting comes with a lot of benefits, it also has its associated downsides, which could either be short term or long term. These effects vary from one individual to another.

Poor weight management. Many people tend to crave for and consume more calories after a long period of fasting, which will inevitably counteract all the progress, made by fasting.

Short-term downsides. Fasting could have several adverse effects such: dizziness, headaches, outbursts, weakness, low blood pressure, and gouts/gall stones among others.

Long-Term downsides. Continuous prolonged fasting could weaken the immune system and affect vital organs such as the kidneys and the liver. When an individual abstains from food over a long period, he becomes malnourished and could lead to an untimely death after the entire energy store of the body has been exhausted.

Dry Fast. Dry fasting is the most dangerous form of fasting in which an individual abstains from food and fluids. It could even lead to death if other underlying factors such as exertions, heat and the likes set in.

Precautions to Take When Fasting

Fasting has a lot of advantages. However, fasting is not meant for everyone. To better understand the theory of fasting, let us compare Fasting to a tool (such as an arrow), which can either be used properly or misused. Holding to that, we will use the archery metaphor to explain the effective use and the misuse of fasting/autophagy. A hunter could have different sizes and tips of arrows in his quiver. When he finds an antelope, he will use a sharp wooden arrow, but when faced by a lion or bear, he would go for something stronger: probably an arrow with metallic tips. The point is don't use the wrong method for the right purpose.

Who should avoid fasting
Pregnant and breastfeeding mothers. Whether you have a child you're breastfeeding or one who is still in your uterus, you need all the calories you can get; both the mother and the infant need to be fed well to stay nourished and healthy.

Underage students and those below 18 should avoid Fasting. Children under the age of 18 are still growing and need all the vital nutrients and minerals to have healthy growth and development.

Those that is underweight and/or malnourished. If you find it difficult to tell whether you are malnourished or not, you could ask your physician or a trusted friend. Those having an eating disorder such as bulimia are included in this category.

Individuals who have Type-2 Diabetes. Fasting has been used over the years as a means of reversing the effect of Type-2 diabetes. However, you still need to consult your physician before beginning a fast.

Who needs to be cautious?
Another group of individuals who also need to be cautious is those with occasional gastroesophageal reflux disease (GERD). Those who fall into this category need to check with their physician as well if they wish to fast and must be closely monitored.

There are solid pieces of evidence to prove that fasting could aggravate GERD and the symptoms could become worsened. This possible worsening is because during fasting, the stomach will be devoid of food and there will be nothing, which the gastric juice would digest.

Individuals on medications need to be cautious while fasting as the fasting periods could overlap when such drugs would be taken especially those medications that would require you to eat before using them.

In addition, those on cancer therapy and other medical treatment must be cautious and should have an in-depth discussion with their physician before fasting.

I have seen a lot of people start with an intermittent fasting plan and end up complaining that the program is not working for them. The same person would then tell me that they do not have a very physical lifestyle.

You should have read the topic where I explained how intermittent fasting is used for weight loss already by now, so you should understand that without expending calories each day, you won't be able to lose that excess fat that has accumulated inside your body.

Expending calories mean being physically active. Unfortunately, quite a large percentage of the worldwide population is living sedentary lifestyles. With a sedentary lifestyle, you are really "paving the way" for weight gain. If you are not physically active, you won't be able to burn an adequate number of calories each day for weight loss to be possible in the first place.

Thus, when you decide to follow my intermittent fasting weight loss cookbook and meal plan, then you should be sure also to include an appropriate exercise plan. Make sure you are physically active according to the prescribed standards – you should be physically active on a few days each week at a minimum.

The more you exercise, the more calories you will burn, of course. At the same time, you should be sure not to overdo things in terms of physical activity. There really is no use in causing you injury due to overtraining – this will only lead to temporary disability and will make training harder for the next few days (sometimes weeks or months if you suffer a more serious injury).

It is best to create a balanced exercise plan for yourself and then test it out. Listen to your body and understand when you are pushing yourself, as well as when you have some extra capacity available to up your game at the gym.

You will have to take your daily calorie consumption into account here – we did discuss how you could calculate your ideal daily calorie requirement in a previous section. This data will definitely come in handy here. Calculate an appropriate exercise plan that will ensure your daily caloric expenditure reached through physical exercise will reach past your daily caloric intake.

So, the question now is, should you give in to the temptations that you will be experiencing, especially during those first few days, or should you implement an appropriate strategy to help you better cope with these hunger pangs and the cravings that you are going to experience.

There are different strategies that you can use to cope with your cravings. One would be to drink a glass of water if you feel hungry and you can feel those cravings building up. This is an effective strategy for lots of people, but not for everyone, of course. If you find that plain water or even filtered water does not work well for you, then I suggest you try some fizzy water (carbonated water). Be sure not to opt for carbonated water with added sweetening agents, as these are loaded with some carbs. Rather just opt for plain sparkling water. The carbonation in the water can help to make you feel full for a while to ensure you can get through to your eating window without giving in to your temptations.

It is important that you are patient and practice self-control when cravings start building up. Giving in to these cravings should not be considered okay now-and-then, as this will break the fasting window and it will yield less effective results compared to ensuring you last until you are inside of your eating window.

Chapter 6: Intermittent Fasting and Heart Health

So far, we have spent some time talking about the amazing benefits that can come with intermittent fasting. We have even talked about some of the ways that fasting can help improve the health of your heart, such as by lowering your cholesterol levels and reducing inflammation. Just by increasing your insulin sensitivity, intermittent fasting can help reduce your risk of heart disease by 93 percent.

When it comes to looking just at the heart and how healthy it is, many experts look at a variety of factors, including inflammatory markers, blood pressure, triglycerides, and cholesterol levels. And it just happens that intermittent fasting can help reduce all these risk factors. Let's look at how intermittent fasting can really help improve your heart health so that you can live a long and happy life.

How Does Intermittent Fasting Help with Circulation and Healthy Hearts?

Intermittent fasting can be very effective at reducing your risk of circulatory and heart disease. Cardiovascular diseases are one of the leading causes of death in the world, with one in six deaths in the United States attributed to heart disease and one in 19 deaths due to a stroke. Many people wrongly assume that heart disease only occurs in men, but women can be just as much, if not more, at risk of this disease.

There are a variety of risk factors that can lead to cardiovascular disease. Some of these include:

- Being overweight. This is particularly concerning if your waistline is larger and you carry more weight around your middle.

- Lack of exercise.
- Poor diet.
- Diabetes.
- Insulin resistance and a high level of glucose in the blood.
- High blood pressure.
- Smoking has been shown to cause several issues with your heart health. The chemicals that are found in cigarettes can easily cause the blood vessels to narrow, forcing the heart to pump blood harder than before.

Fasting can help with some of these risk factors. For example, it can help you to lose weight so that your weight and your waistline are no longer a big issue. It can help lower your blood pressure, reduce the risk that you have for diabetes, and can reduce insulin resistance. Fasting can even help you get on a healthier diet because your cravings for processed and junk foods will be reduced. If you add in a healthy lifestyle to this as well, you may be able to stop smoking and add in more exercise to help with those risk factors as well.

A Look at How Cardiovascular Disease Can Develop

Cardiovascular disease is a pretty general term that is used to discuss all of the diseases that can occur to your circulation and your heart. It can include coronary heart disease, like a heart attack or angina, heart failure, and even stroke. These diseases are all going to be caused when fatty deposits are allowed to build up in the arteries, a process that is known as atherosclerosis.

The exact cause of this is not always certain. Many people originally thought that it was obvious that having higher levels of fat in the blood would be the culprit of this issue. However, scientific research has shown that this is too easy, and it may not always be the case. The exact kinds of fats that you consume will be the important part. In addition, the amount of inflammation that is found in the arteries may be a factor as well. Carrying an excess amount of fat around the internal organs and having issues with resistance to insulin can also increase your risk of developing this condition.

What is known is that once fats build up in the arteries, they become narrower and stiffer. The result of this is an increase in your blood pressure because it takes more pressure to get the blood through your narrowed arteries. If this narrowing occurs too much, then there can be a problem like angina, pain when walking, and even heart attacks. The heart is working hard to pump blood throughout the body, but if the arteries get completely blocked, then the organs, including the heart, won't be able to get the blood that they need to function.

This kind of health concern is going to occur over time, with an unhealthy lifestyle and diet. Many people may not realize the extent of their issues and will wait until it is too late to do something that will make it better. It is much better to work on a healthier lifestyle and diet as early as possible to ensure that you don't have to deal with any of the many cardiovascular diseases that can harm your body.

Is Intermittent Fasting Able to Reduce My Risk of Developing Cardiovascular Disease?

The good news is that many studies have found that intermittent fasting can improve the risk factors for cardiovascular disease. This means that when you are on a fast, you can reduce your risks of developing one of these diseases. Some risk factors, such as insulin resistance, cholesterol, blood pressure, and weight (particularly fat that is around your waist), can all be improved with intermittent fasting.

Individuals who went on a 24-hour fast just once a month were less likely to be diagnosed with coronary artery disease. This is based on a study of 448 people in Utah and those who fasted that was also suffering from type 2 diabetes. Imagine the changes that could happen if these individuals chose to fast for more than one day a month, such as doing the 5:2 diets or an alternate day fasting schedule. Their risk of developing cardiovascular disease may be even lower.

In addition, there were studies done on obese and overweight women who were asked to fast every other day for eight weeks. These participants were allowed to have about 500 calories a day on their fasting day. After the eight weeks were over, these women had lost weight and reduced their waist size, decreased their LDL and cholesterol, lowered their blood pressure, and more.

In a further study, it was found that these same kinds of improvements to cardiovascular health were also seen in people whether they ate on the traditional diet most Americans follow or a low-fat diet on their non-fasting days. Moreover, other studies that look at alternate day fasting have confirmed these benefits to the health of your heart.

Another research study showed that overweight women who did a semi-fast for two days a week, which meant they could eat up to 600 calories on their fasting days, had a reduction in insulin resistance, blood pressure, triglycerides, total and LDL cholesterol, inflammation, and leptin. This shows that whether the women went on an alternate day fast or the 5:2 diets, they saw results that could improve the health of their heart.

Studies have also been done on daily fasting during Ramadan. These studies show that there was an improvement in cardiovascular risks with this type of fasting as well. Often, this form of fasting is not going to be used for the health benefits, though, and is done to follow a religion. Some studies may not encourage this form of fasting to keep you healthy for the long term.

To get some of the good benefits that come from intermittent fasting, you must take the time to eat a diet that is healthy and wholesome. If you go on one of these fasting choices and then spend your time eating a lot of junk and processed foods, it isn't going to help your risk of developing cardiovascular disease, and you will be in just as much trouble as before.

The exact way that intermittent fasting can cause beneficial changes to your cardiovascular risk is still unknown. However, it seems like some of the key factors include helping the individual to lose weight, improve their insulin resistance, and inflammation. The reduction in waist size can be a good indicator that you are heading in the right direction when it comes to reducing your risk of cardiovascular disease. If you have a large risk for cardiovascular disease or you have some of the risk factors discussed above, then it may be time to consider going on a 5:2 diet or an alternate day fast to help you get some results to cut down on your cardiovascular risk.

Motivation for you While Intermittent Fasting

It is understood that it is not always easy to stay on a diet. Although the intermittent fast cannot be thought of as a diet, it requires you to make lifestyle and food choices that can be a little taxing at times.

In this chapter, we will look at simple things that you can do to stick with the fast.

Expectations

It is obvious that you will have a lot of expectations from the diet. It is normal to have them, as you will want to reach your ideal weight within a certain period of time. But what is important to note is that you have to have realistic expectations when it comes to the time frame you set to achieve the weight loss. You cannot achieve it overnight. If you are obese now, then try to go for a 6 to 12-month plan to lose weight. If you go for something lesser then it might not work out for you. If you set an unrealistic goal and see that it is not working out for you then you will feel discouraged and might want to go off the diet. It is therefore important to set realistic goals in order to achieve them better.

Motivators

Make sure you know exactly why you are going for the weight loss routine. It is obvious that you will want to lose weight and fit into smaller clothes etc. But apart from these, there have to be other motivators as well that will keep you on track. Make a list of them and stick them in your room or have a copy of the list on your phone so that you can look at it and remain motivated. These will keep you from going for something unhealthy and sticking with the fast.

Clear out the kitchen

A top tip is to get rid of all junk and processed foods from the kitchen. These can be quite tempting. Follow the rule, "out of sight, out of mind." Go through everything in the kitchen and get rid of all items that are bad for the diet. Keep it off the shelves and off the counters. Replace them with healthier alternatives such as nuts. Make sure you do not go into the kitchen after a certain point in time say 10 or 11 at night. Once you have had your last meal, stay away from the kitchen area. If you have a lot of junk and processed food lying around then throw a party to finish it all in one go.

Don't be too harsh

Don't be too harsh on yourself if you end up going for a cheat meal. It can be a little difficult to make a sudden change in your lifestyle. It is therefore advisable to go slow with it. Make sure you ease into the diet so that you can stave off temptations. Do not be tempted to fall off the wagon just because you had one cheat meal. Treat it as a cheat and focus on your fast.

Carry your food

Do not forget to carry your meals everywhere you go. Be it to the office or to a party, you have to carry the meals with you so that you can avoid the hassle of settling for something that is forbidden by the diet. If you don't have a ready snack with you then you are bound to go for something unhealthy. Have a high-protein snack ready that you can bite into as soon as you get hungry. A few good options include peanuts, almonds and a hard-boiled egg. These can keep you going until the next meal.

Don't go for too much

If you are just starting out with the fast then make sure you go slowly. Do not do too many things at once, as that will confuse your body. If you do not exercise at all then go for simple ones at first. Once you have settled into the diet, go for an exercise routine. If you start both at once then you will do justice to neither. But make sure at some point you take up exercising and do not rely on the fast alone. It would be best to wait for about a month before taking up an exercise regime. Although research suggests you have to stick to something for at least a month for the habit to stick, it is best you take it up seriously and continue for at least 6 months to a year.

Do your research

It is obvious that in this day and age nobody can go without eating out. It can be quite a challenge to go out and not find something edible on the menu. In such a case, it pays to do your research and make sure you find a restaurant that serves meals that cater to your choice. It will be even better if you find something that customizes the menu for you. If you are traveling, then plan ahead and find out which places you can eat at. Pack enough food to keep you going for at least 3 days. Make sure you go for foods that can last at least a week.

Reward yourself

It is always important to reward yourself with something nice for keeping up the good work. It can be a trip to the spa or a vacation. You can also buy yourself something that you have always wanted like a crock-pot or an air fryer. A recipe book too can serve as a reward. The reward can be anything as long as you feel motivated to keep up with the diet. It would be advisable not to go for a cheat meal as a reward.

Mindfulness and meditation

Mindfulness is a technique that helps you dig deep into your thoughts and remain completely focused on the task at hand. By practicing mindful eating, you give yourself the chance to enjoy a healthy meal. Those who enjoy their meals are able to better connect with the food and lose a significant amount of weight just by remaining focused on the meal. Another research found that mindfulness successfully put an end to binge eating. It is said to have reduced from almost 4 to 1.5 times a week over a period of 6 weeks. It is, therefore, a good idea to indulge in mindfulness eating. You can also engage in meditation. This can keep your mind calm. Try to stay away from stress as much as possible as it can negatively impact your health. It can also cause you to gain weight. The more stress free you remain, the better off you are in terms of attaining weight loss.

Keep track

Keep track of your progress. This can serve as a big motivator to keep you on track. Maintain a diary and write down everything including your weight, measurements, meal timings, meal plans, etc. Refer back to it from time to time to ensure that you are on the right track. It is a good idea to maintain a blog and keep updating your progress. Your friends and family members can access it and encourage you to keep up the good work.

Partner up

Getting a partner is always a great way to remain motivated to stick to a fast. Not only will you have company, you will also remain motivated to keep t it. It can be a spouse, partner, sibling, colleague, friend, etc., as long as they wish to benefit from the fast. Usually, when one partner decides to make a healthy choice be it dietary modification or exercise, the other decides to follow as well. You will also find it easier with your partner chipping in to prepare the healthy meals and keeping track of your progress.

Go for a heavy breakfast

There is nothing better than a healthy and hearty breakfast or rather the first meal of the day. If you plan on having your meal by 12 noon then go for something that is loaded with proteins and other nutrients. As per studies, women who ate 1.05 ounces of protein for breakfast were able to avoid feeling puckish before lunch as compared to those who ate a breakfast low in proteins. You can also have a protein and fiber rich lunch to supplement the breakfast.

Take your time

Don't be in a hurry to get through everything at once. Go about it in a slow and steady manner. As mentioned earlier, it might take at least a month for you to make a habit stick. Be patient with it. Keep at it for at least 6 months. Do not compare yourself to others. If there are people passing negative comments, then learn to ignore them. You have to remain focused and motivated to achieve the slimmer, fitter and better you.

Customize

Customize the diet for yourself. Only you will know your body best. Do not follow what someone else is following as what works for him or her might not work for you. It is best to come up with a plan that is sustainable in the long run as compared to one that will only provide you momentary results.

These are just some of the things you can do to remain motivated. Do not limit it to just these and do whatever it takes for you to stick with the intermittent fast.

Chapter 7: What to Eat While Intermittent Fasting

In this chapter, we will look at some of the foods that you simply must include in your diet while you take up the fast.

Water

This is definitely the most important element to consume when you take up the intermittent fast. Water can act as an elixir when it comes to losing weight. You must keep your body hydrated and ensure that all the toxins are dissolved and eliminated. All your organs need water to remain fresh and healthy; right from your liver to gut to digestive tract, water helps to keep these organs working smoothly. Drink at least 8 to 10 glasses of water a day and focus more on the fasting period. It is obvious that it will get a little monotonous and so, a good idea is to consume fruit infused water. This refers to water that has fruit and herbs infused into it. Fill up a jar with water and toss in fruit and herbs such as oranges, lemons, mint leaves and a dash of cinnamon. Consume this every few hours. Remember that the intermittent fast can be quite taxing at times and lead to side effects such as headache and nausea. In such a case, only water can help you out and put an end to these.

Fish

Fish can be considered as a miracle food as it can greatly help with weight loss. According to dietary guidelines, it is important for people to consume at least 6 to 8 ounces of fish every week. Fish contains a lot of nutrients. It is rich in fats and proteins. It is also rich in vitamin D. and this means you do not have to worry about denying your body these nutrients by taking on the fast. You do not have to reach for supplements if you are able to consume fish regularly. Fish is also rich in DHA, which helps in brain development. You will see that your mind is fresher and you are able to think well. Your productivity will increase and stress will be curbed.

Avocado

You might wonder why avocado is in this list considering it is one of the fattiest foods out there. However, you must understand that the fasting phase can take a toll on your body and so you must consume foods that can keep you going. Avocado is rich in monounsaturated fat, which is great for those who tend to get hungry quite fast. It keeps you feeling full for longer. You will not find yourself reaching out to eat a snack. Avocado is quite versatile and can be added to your breakfast or lunch menu. Those who tend to include it in their breakfast menu are generally able to go without food for longer periods of time without complaining about hunger.

Leafy greens

If there is one type of vegetable that we remember being told to consume by our parents then it has to be leafy green vegetables. As we know, leafy green vegetables are loaded with multiple nutrients that are great for your body. These include the likes of kale, broccoli, lettuce, etc. These are loaded with fiber. Fiber, as you know, keeps your body going when you suffer from digestive issues such as constipation. You are sure to go through it when you adopt the intermittent fast. In such a case, it becomes that much more important to consume these vegetables to keep your stomach in good shape. Fiber also makes you feel fuller and not feel too hungry between meals.

Potatoes

As mentioned earlier, the goal is to consume foods that are filling and can keep you going for hours, one such being potatoes. Potatoes are rich in carbs that can keep you sated for hours. Make sure you either steam and mash them or roast them without the addition of any oil or fat. Deep frying them is never an option. Try to consume them with their skin on as the skin contains a lot of nutrition.

Probiotics

When it comes to digestion, both your liver and gut play a very important role. Both of them need a healthy dose of probiotics in order to function optimally. If you have an unhealthy gut then you might suffer from side effects such as constipation and even leaky gut syndrome. The best way to combat these is by consuming as many probiotics as possible. Some natural foods rich in probiotics include kombucha and kefir. Add these to your meals and you are sure to experience positive benefits. An alternative is to go for probiotic supplements. Make sure you know which ones to go for. It would be best to consult a physician first.

Assorted berries

There is nothing better than consuming fresh berries in the mornings. They are loaded with antioxidants and vital nutrients required to keep your body healthy. Strawberries, raspberries, blueberries and gooseberries all are great for you. Just toss them into the blender with some milk or yogurt to make a smoothie. According to studies, those who consumed berries regularly were able to remain within their ideal body weight and did not gain too much weight over longer periods of time.

Eggs

An important aspect of losing weight is building lean muscles. Lean muscles replace regular ones and prevent fat from getting stored. The best way to build lean muscle is by consuming foods rich in proteins. One important source of proteins is eggs. Those who consume eggs for breakfast are in a better position to develop lean muscles and not go hungry before the next meal. Eggs can be quite versatile and cooked in any way you like. Hard-boil them the previous day so that you have a ready meal the next morning. Simply toss them in a pan to scramble them. It only takes a few minutes to cook them.

Whole grains

One aspect of maintaining a clean and healthy diet is going for whole grains. The intermittent fast promotes consumption of these, as they are easier for the body to digest and keep the system clean. They are also loaded with proteins and fiber. Do not limit yourself to the usual such as wheat and oats and go for something different such as Bulgar, amaranth and flax.

Legumes

If you wish to remain full for longer and not feel hungry or peckish too often then there is nothing better than legumes and beans. These cannot only be quite flavorful but also loaded with fiber. The body does not easily digest fiber. In fact, the body cannot digest it at all but makes extra effort in trying to digest it thereby drawing into the fat reserves. It is, therefore, best to load up on fiber in order to lose weight easily. There are many options to pick from including peas, lentils, green beans, fava, black-eyed peas, etc. These easily fit into soups and salads.

Nuts

Nuts are fatty no doubt, but they contain good fat. Not all fat is bad fat as there can be some good fat as well. Polyunsaturated fats are said to be good for the body and can keep you feeling full for longer. You will not feel hungry if you munch on some walnuts or almonds. But make sure you make them a part of your meal and do not snack on them. Snacking on them can leave you feeling full and disrupt your meal plan. Do not worry about the calorie aspect. Nuts are not as calorific as you may have thought. They contain far less calories than some of the other fatty foods that people tend to snack on.

These happen to be superfoods that you must include in your diet while you take up intermittent fasting.

Foods to Avoid While Intermittent Fasting

Processed foods

Processed foods include the likes of biscuits, wafers, chips, cakes and sugary drinks such as cola. These will only add to your woes and counteract your weight loss goals. Try to avoid these at all costs. Do not hit the aisles at the supermarket that carry these foods. Remember to never go shopping on an empty stomach, as you will feel tempted to reach for a packet or snack.

Junk foods

Make it a point to cut out all junk food from your diet. There should be no room for burgers, pizzas and pastas that contain a lot of fat. It might be tempting to go for a cheat meal once in a while, but it is important not to do so as it can lead to a habit.

Alcohol

Although wine is said to be quite healthy, it would be best to limit it to just 1 serving per week. Try your best to avoid consuming hard liquor.

Although it is said that the intermittent fast does not tell you what not to eat, it is best to avoid these when you wish to lose weight.

With intermittent fasting, a lot of people tend to follow their usual eating habits in terms of the specific foods that they put on their plate during each meal, expecting that they will lose weight just because they have fasted during the morning, night, and a part of the afternoon.

While intermittent fasting may help to improve metabolism and support digestive function that will ultimately improve your ability to lose weight, the food you eat still counts. As you might have noted, the meal plans that I shared with you in this cookbook generally combines a range of healthy foods in order to ensure you get the nutrients you need without loading up on too many carbs. I did include a lot of delicious options that you can try out.

Just as there are a lot of foods that you can surely include in your diet to help you lose that extra weight that is causing you concern, there are also some foods that you should always try to avoid if your goal is to lose weight.

Below, I would like to share some of the most important foods that you should try to exclude from your diet in order to improve the results you are able to achieve when you implement the recipes and meal plans I have provided you within this book.

- Fried foods, of course, should be at the top of my list. There is no doubt that fried foods are one particularly common reason for the world to be so obese. Millions of people eat fried foods as much as every day. This does not only cause them to gain in weight, but also to experience a rise in cholesterol levels, be at a higher risk of heart disease, and more.

- Fast foods, along with fried foods, since most chains that offer fast foods tend to deep fry their food in the worst types of oil and fat to make them more 'tasty' for the general public. Unfortunately, this also adds more fat to your belly, thighs, arms, and other areas of your body.

- Corn is another food that really isn't the best choice for people who are trying to lose weight. Sure, it is not an unhealthy food, but consider the fact that this is a type of grain that is relatively high in sugar. The sugar spike experienced when you eat corn leads to the release of insulin, triggering inflammation and taking you one step closer to the dreadful complications of insulin resistance.

In addition to all of these, be sure to be wary of added sugars in everything you eat. For example, if you visit your local supermarket and grab a healthy bar to use as the food to break your fast, the fact that the word "healthy" appears on the bar does not necessarily mean it is truly healthy.

Always look at the ingredients of what you buy and what you will be putting into your body. Making your own healthy energy bars at home might be a better solution as well.

Chapter 8: Example Meal Plan for Weight Loss with Intermittent Fasting

If you do a quick search on Google for a weight loss plan that you can use with intermittent fasting, you will be surprised at just how many variations there are that you can choose from. This can really make the entire process challenging, instead of a fun and exciting journey that you are taking on in order to help you achieve a body that you will feel more confident about.

Many of the weight loss plans available can be effective if you stick to the plan and you ensure your body is provided with an adequate amount of exercise on a daily basis. Unfortunately, this does not make it easier to choose one that is ideal for you.

Below, we will take a look at an example of a really good intermittent fasting diet plan that you can follow and adjust according to your own preferences and requirements if you are finding it hard to choose an appropriate option for yourself. This is a very basic "framework" that you can work from.

Before we look at the example weight loss intermittent fasting meal plan – there is one thing that you should note. DO not expect everything to go smoothly the first time around. On your first few days, know that things can be rather difficult. This is especially true if you are used to eating continuously during the day – which is a very common problem among people who have a more significant amount of weight to lose.

Be patient in the beginning – with yourself and with the results you achieve through your diet plan. After a week or two, if you do not see the results that you expect, then aim to make a few adjustments in order to customize your diet plan and your intermittent fasting program to be more appropriate to your goals.

With the diet plan example that I am about to share with you – I want you to get into a habit of skipping breakfast. With the 16/8 programs, you will only have a window between six to eight hours where you will consume food every day. Since you are aiming to lose weight, skipping out on breakfast means your body will start to utilize its own fat reserves in order to generate energy. This is ideal for someone who needs to lose weight.

You will have your first meal at 3 pm in the afternoon. Have your second meal at around 6 pm and then finish off the day with a final meal at around 10 pm.

Your first two meals of the day should be kept light. This way, you won't turn off your body's automatic fat burning mechanisms. By the end of the day, you'll consume a meal that is heavier on the calorie side. Even though you are free to experiment with the number of calories you consume during each meal, be wary of what food you decide to consume – you are trying to lose weight and become a healthier person. For this reason, always ensure that you eat healthily as well.

I personally recommend that the first two meals of your day should be a maximum of 400 calories each. Be sure that there is an adequate supply of protein in these meals. Don't skim on vegetables and fruits – enjoy them, as they are good for you.

Here are some examples of small and light meals that you may wish to experiment with for your first two meals (at 3 pm and at 6 pm):

- Add some almonds and a couple of berries into a cup of Greek yogurt.

- Have some cottage cheese with a couple of almonds.

- Add one tablespoon of olive oil to a can of tuna, and enjoy your meal with an apple.

- Use two whole eggs to make yourself an omelet. Have this meal with some delicious berries.

If you are in the mood for a meatier meal, then cook up a chicken breast and enjoy it with a green salad. You can add half of an Avocado to the meal, as well as an apple.

For those who are in a hurry and would like to drink something instead, mixing a cup of unsweetened almond milk with about 40 grams of whey protein powder is a really good option. You can have some fruit with this, as well as about 20 grams of almonds.

When it comes to the third meal of the day – this is when you should enter the kitchen and prepare something healthy and delicious-tasting for yourself. There are a lot of different healthy meals that you can choose to fill the gap at 10 pm. It is a good idea to limit the last meal of the day to around 800 calories, but you can push it up to around 1000 calories if you wish.

When it comes to your last meal, it is important to balance fats and protein perfectly to avoid weight gain or other potential side-effects from your diet plan. If you are opting for a leaned piece of meat (to supply your body with quality protein), then you can have more healthy types of fats in your meal. If, on the other hand, you decide to opt for a fattier type of meal, let's say a piece of beefsteak that is a fatty cut, then you should limit how much-added fats you put into your meal.

To help you prepare your third and final meal of the day, here are three examples of meals that are nutritious and will give you that final amount of calories that you need during your eating window:

- Cook up a chicken breast and serve it with some potato wedges and a variety of vegetables.

- Serve some brown rice with vegetables and a chicken breast. Try to use a small amount of coconut oil to cook both the rice and the chicken.

- If you are rather in the mood for some beef, then have a steak with some vegetables. You can also serve this up with a sweet potato – add a little bit of cinnamon to the sweet potato for additional flavor.

Exercising with Intermittent Fasting

Ask anyone who had successful results with any type of dieting program in the past – and they would tell you that exercise was a crucial part of their weight loss program. The primary idea behind any type of diet that aims to help you reduce your body weight is to create a caloric deficit.

Thus, when you are implementing a diet plan along with intermittent fasting to help you lose weight, then you should ensure that you also implement an appropriate exercise program.

Some people are concerned about exercising while following a program that utilizes intermittent fasting strategies. However, once your body is used to this new eating style, you'll notice that it becomes easier and easier. There are also a variety of supplements that you can take to boost your endurance and stamina and to give you that extra energy that you will need to ensure you can get past a training session, even while you are fasting.

Here's a little-known secret that many people do not realize in terms of exercising while you are on an intermittent fasting program: the fat burning mechanisms of the human body is regulated by what is known as the sympathetic nervous system. This system is also called the SNS for short. When the system activates, it means your body starts to burn fat. There are two essential elements that cause the SNS system to activate – this includes a lack of food in your body, as well as exercise. When you decide to give your body a dose of both, then activation is more thorough, and your SNS will lead to a much more significant level of fat burning and weight loss.

There are many other benefits that should be taken into account in terms of exercising while you are fasting. One particular benefit that becomes especially useful for those people who are trying to bulk up with muscle mass while they are following a plan that uses intermittent fasting is the fact that exercising during your fast window will cause oxidative stress. While oxidative stress is often considered a bad thing for the body, during exercise, it can actually be good for improving your muscle strength and mass.

Take this into account as well – if you eat before you participate in an exercise program, then there is a chance that the food you consumed may lead to issues with your general performance during your routine. It has been found that the consumption of food in any form – be it a shake, an energy bar, or an actual meal – causes your blood glucose levels to experience a spike while you are exercising. Sure, this will give you some energy to kick start that tough routine that you are about to start – but, once this spike is over, your blood glucose levels will quickly decline, and you will basically experience a "crash." What this means is you will feel the fatigue coming on quickly, leading to poor muscle performance and a body that is quickly running out of energy.

There are, however, some publications that say this is a myth – but this is still something that you should consider when it comes to intermittent fasting!

All in all, there are a specific number of benefits that you may expect from a good workout program integrated into your intermittent fasting plan. You will be able to experience the following potential benefits with this particular combination:

- You can turn back what is known as the "biological clock" on your brain, as well as your muscles, due to the effects of exercise on your body while in a fasting state.

- The concentration of growth hormone produced by your body will be increased.

- Your body composition will be greatly improved, as you will experience a reduction in body fat percentage, along with an increase in lean muscle mass.

- Cognitive function will also benefit, and you'll find that problems like brain fog start to disappear.

- Your testosterone levels are likely to rise as well, which can be especially beneficial for older men who are experiencing a natural decline in the level of circulating testosterone within their bodies.

While exercising while fasting is definitely beneficial for you and your weight, there is one particular factor that I have to mention here. On days when you are going to do some heavy lifting as part of your exercise routine, it is crucial that you get your timing right. When you decide to participate in some heavy lifting exercises, then you will need to ensure you eat something within the first 30 minutes after you have completed the heavy lifting workout.

Chapter 9: Recipes

Breakfast

Breakfast Quiche

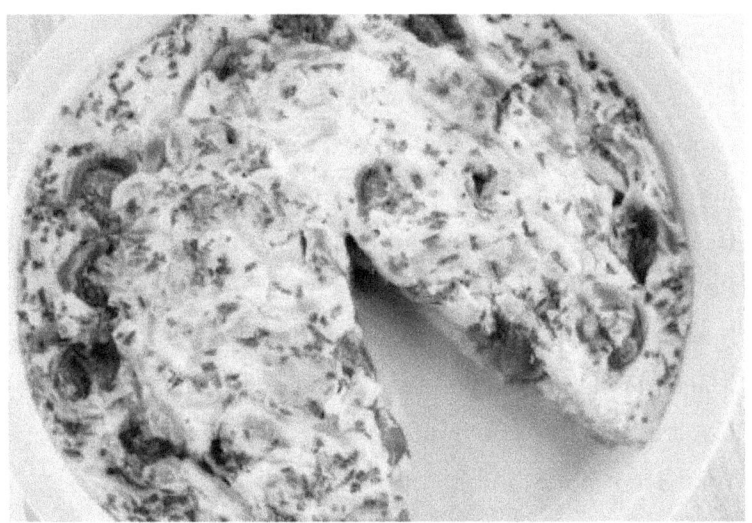

Total time: 35 minutes
Servings: 3

Ingredients

- Diced tomatoes – ½ cup
- Chopped spinach – 1 ½ cups
- Grated Parmesan cheese – 2 tbsp.
- Almond milk – ¼ cup
- Green onions – 1 ½, chopped
- Eggs – 6

- Tomato – ½, sliced
- Garlic salt – ¼ tsp.
- Pepper to taste
- Water – 1 ½ cups

Method

1. Pour the water into the IP.
2. Grease a baking dish with cooking spray.
3. Combine the green onions, diced tomatoes, and spinach in it.
4. Beat the eggs along with salt, pepper, and milk.
5. Pour this mixture over the spinach and tomatoes.
6. Sprinkle with Parmesan cheese and top with tomato slices.
7. Place the baking dish on the rack and close the lid.
8. Cook on High for 20 minutes.
9. Wait 10 minutes before releasing the pressure quickly.
10. Serve.

Nutritional Facts Per Serving
- Calories: 178
- Fat: 11.2g
- Carb: 3.8g
- Protein: 15.3g

Avocado Eggs Stir-Fry

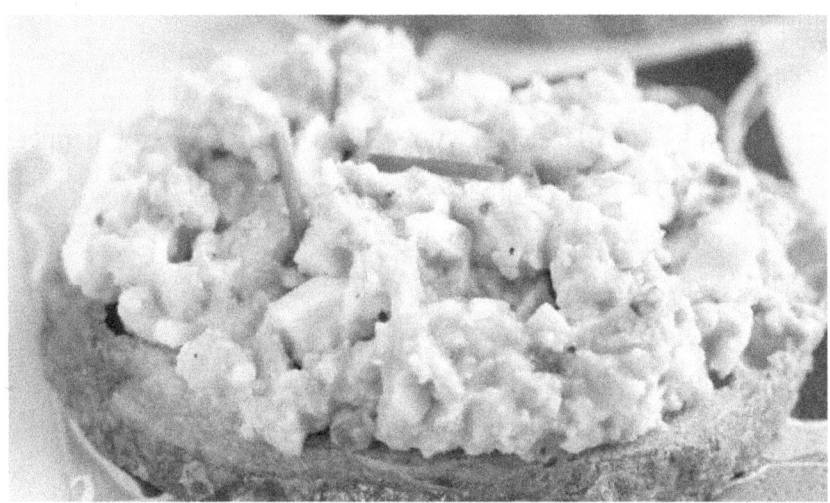

Total time: 15 minutes
Servings: 2

Ingredients
- Medium avocado – 1, pitted and cubed
- Large eggs – 2, beaten
- Green onions – 2 tbsp. finely chopped
- Olive oil – 1 tsp.
- Butter – 1 tbsp.
- Plain Greek yogurt or heavy cream for serving to taste

Spices:

- Sea salt – ½ tsp.
- Black pepper – ¼ tsp. ground

- Red chili flakes – ¼ tsp.

Method

1. Melt the butter in your IP over the Sauté setting.
2. Add avocado cubes and season with salt and pepper. Cook for 3 to 4 minutes, stirring occasionally.
3. Now, add the green onions, eggs, and olive oil.
4. Cook until the eggs are set, about 3 minutes more. Press the Cancel and turn off the pot.
5. Transfer to serving plates.
6. Serve topped with heavy cream or plain Greek yogurt.
7. Enjoy.

Nutritional Facts Per Serving
- Calories: 350
- Fat: 32.7g
- Carb: 2.6g
- Protein: 8.4g

Almond Porridge

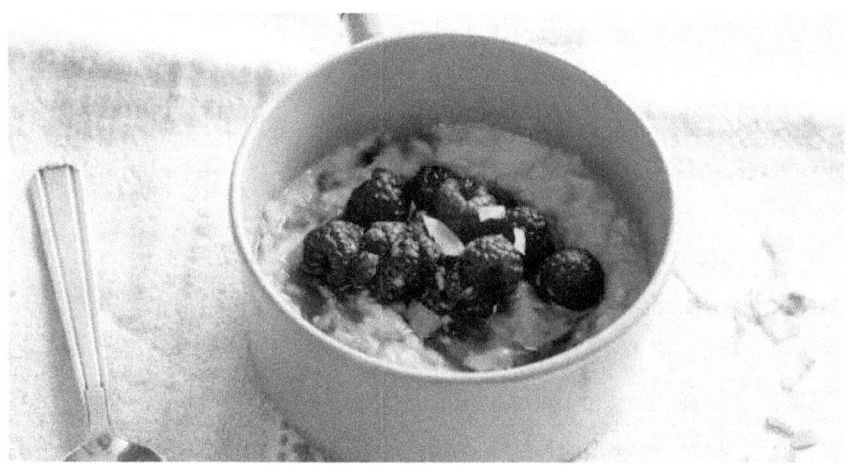

Total time: 10 minutes

Servings: 2

Ingredients

- Unsweetened almond milk - 1 cup

- Coconut oil – 3 tbsp.

- Hemp seeds – 3 tbsp.

- Chia seeds – 2 tbsp.

- Water – ½ cup

- Fresh raspberries, for topping

Spices

- Swerve – 1 tsp.
- Vanilla extract – 1 tsp.
- Salt – ¼ tsp.

Method

1. Grease the inner pot of the IP with coconut oil.
2. Add chia and hemp seeds.
3. Pour in ½ cup water and press Sauté.
4. Cook for 5 minutes, stirring constantly.
5. Now pour in the almond milk and sprinkle with swerve, vanilla and salt.
6. Stir well and cook for 5 minutes more.
7. Press Cancel and transfer the porridge to a serving bowl.
8. Top with fresh raspberries and serve.

Nutritional Facts Per Serving
- Calories: 380
- Fat: 37.4g
- Carb: 2.3g
- Protein: 11g

Prosciutto Eggs with Heavy Cream

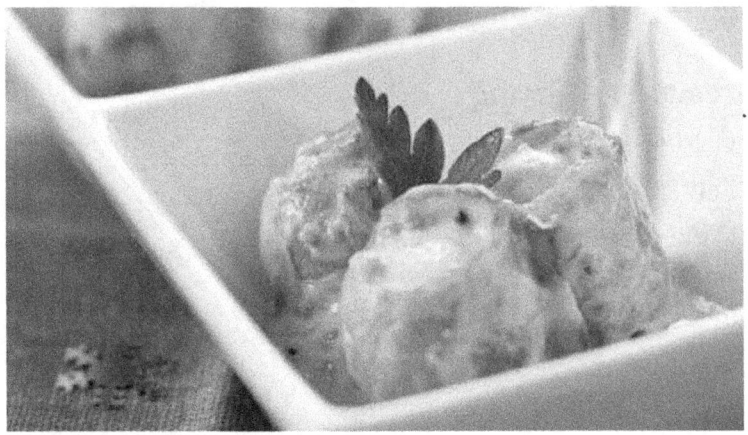

Total time: 15 minutes
Servings: 4

Ingredients

- Kale leaves – 4
- Prosciutto slices – 4
- Heavy cream – 3 tbsp.
- Hardboiled eggs – 4
- Pepper – ¼ tsp.
- Salt to taste
- Water – 1 ½ cup

Method

1. Peel the eggs and wrap them in kale.
2. Wrap them in prosciutto and sprinkle with salt and pepper.
3. Pour the water into the IP and lower the trivet.
4. Place the eggs inside and close the lid.

5. Cook on Manual for 5 minutes.
6. Open the lid and remove.
7. Serve with heavy cream.

Nutritional Facts Per Serving

- Calories: 250
- Fat: 21g
- Carb: 3.2g
- Protein: 15g

Eggs with Ham

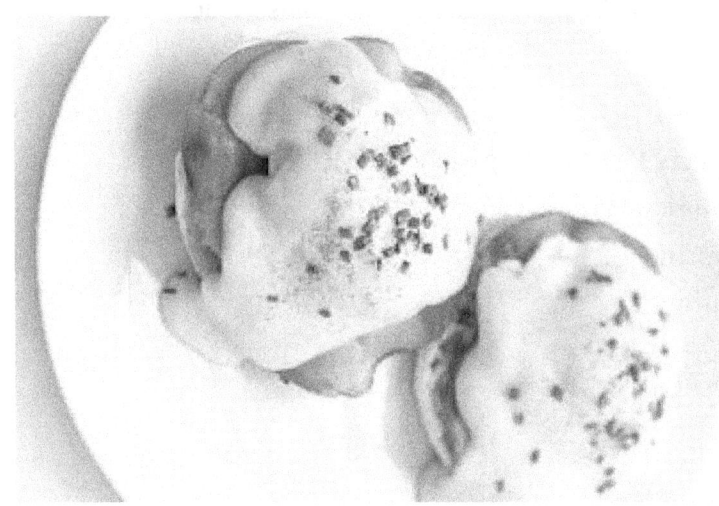

Total time: 10 minutes
Servings: 2

Ingredients
- Eggs – 2
- Hollandaise sauce – 2 tbsp.
- Ham slices – 2, chopped
- Water – 1 ½ cups plus 2 tbsp.

Method

1. Pour 1 ½ cups water into your IP and lower the rack.
2. Crack the egg into 2 ramekins. Make sure to keep the yolks intact.
3. Add 1 tbsp. of water on top.

4. Place the ramekins in the IP and close the lid.
5. Cook on Steam for 2 to 3 minutes.
6. Top with chopped ham and hollandaise sauce.
7. Serve.

Nutritional Facts Per Serving
- Calories: 271
- Fat: 16.2g
- Carb: 5.2g
- Protein: 25.3g

Cauliflower and Sausage Egg Pie

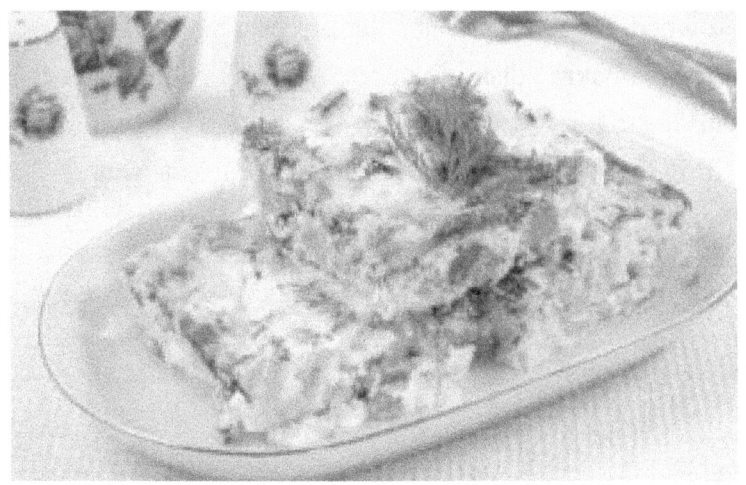

Total time: 30 minutes

Servings: 3

Ingredients

- Eggs – 4, beaten
- Dried basil – 1 tsp.
- Onion – ½, diced
- Cauliflower rice – 1 cup
- Pork sausage – ½ pound
- Garlic powder – ½ tsp.
- Pinch of cumin
- Pinch of turmeric
- Pinch of pepper
- Water – 1 ½ cups

Method

1. Add the sausage in the IP and cook on Sauté until browned. Break it up in smaller pieces while cooking.
2. Grease a baking dish with cooking spray and transfer the sausage to it.
3. Stir in the remaining ingredients, except for the water.
4. Pour the water into the IP and lower the trivet.
5. Place the dish inside and close the IP.
6. Cook on High for 15 to 20 minutes.
7. Do a quick release.
8. Serve.

Nutritional Facts Per Serving

- Calories: 353
- Fat: 26g
- Carb: 5.1g
- Protein: 22g

Breakfast Bagels

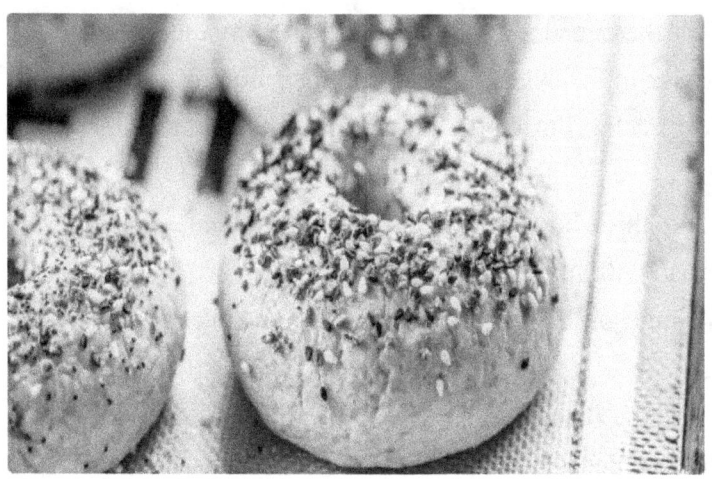

Total time: 30 minutes

Servings: 3

Ingredients
- Almond flour – ¾ cup
- Grated mozzarella cheese – 1 ½ cups.
- Egg – 1
- Cream cheese – 2 tbsp.
- Xanthan gum – ½ tsp.
- Pinch of sea salt
- Water – 1 ½ cups
- Butter – 1 tbsp. melted
- Seeds to top, optional

Method

1. Pour the water into the Instant Pot or IP.
2. Beat the egg along with the xanthan gum and salt.
3. Whisk in the cheeses and stir in the flour.
4. Form a log out of the dough and divide into three equal pieces.
5. Make three bagel-like rings and flatten them.
6. Brush with butter and top with seeds.
7. Arrange on a greased baking tray and place on the IP's rack.
8. Close the lid and cook on Manual for 15 minutes.
9. Release the pressure quickly.
10. Serve and enjoy.

Nutritional Facts Per Serving

- Calories: 367
- Fat: 29g
- Carb: 3.5g
- Protein: 20g

Lunch

<u>Lemon-Garlic Prawns</u>

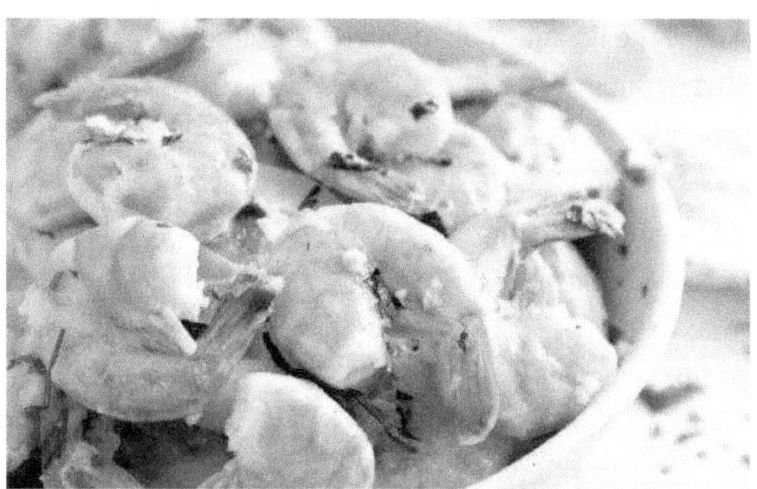

Total time: 15 minutes

Servings: 4

Ingredients

- Minced garlic – 2 tbsp.
- Olive oil – 2 tbsp.
- Lemon zest – 2 tbsp.
- Lemon juice – 2 tbsp.
- Ghee – 1 tbsp.
- Prawns – 1 pound
- Fish stock – 2/3 cup
- Salt and pepper to taste

Method

1. Melt the ghee along with the oil in the Instant Pot on Sauté.
2. Add the remaining ingredients and stir to combine.
3. Close the lid and cook on High for 3 minutes.
4. Drain the prawns.
5. Serve.

Nutritional Facts Per Serving

- Calories: 160
- Fat: 2g
- Carb: 2g
- Protein: 18g

Coconut Milk Cod

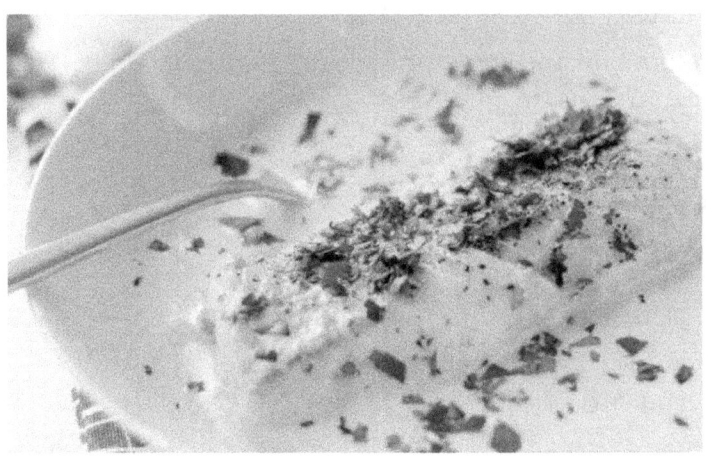

Total time: 20 minutes

Servings: 4

Ingredients

- Cod fillets – 1 pound
- Almond flour – 3 tbsp.
- Lime zest – 1 tbsp.
- Minced garlic – 1 tsp.
- Butter – 1 tbsp.
- Liquid aminos – 2 tbsp.
- Fish sauce – ¼ cup (no sugar added)
- Coconut milk – ½ cup

Method

1. Chop the cod and insert in the IP.
2. Add the remaining ingredients and stir to combine.

3. Set the IP to Sauté and close the lid.
4. Let cook on sauté with the lid on, for about 10 minutes.
5. Open the lid and cook for 3 more minutes.
6. Serve.

Nutritional Facts Per Serving
- Calories: 260
- Fat: 14g
- Carb: 6.1g
- Protein: 24g

Cauliflower and Tomatoes

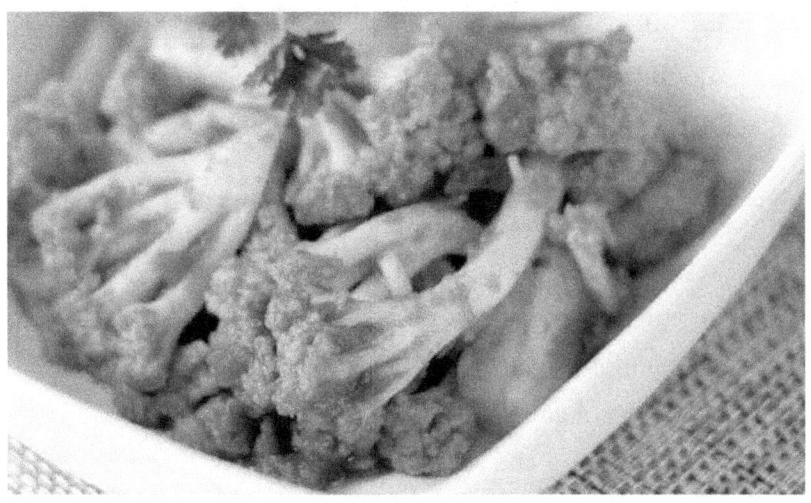

Total time: 22 minutes
Servings: 4

Ingredients
- Chopped tomatoes – 2
- Chopped small onion – ½
- Green chilli – 1
- Olive oil – 1 tsp.
- Ground cumin – 1 tsp.
- Ground turmeric – ½ tsp.
- Paprika – ½ tsp.
- Salt and freshly ground black pepper to taste
- Cauliflower head – 1, cut into small florets
- Water – ½ cup
- Chopped fresh cilantro – 1 tbsp.

Method

1. Add the onion, tomato, and green chili to a food processor and pulse until smooth.
2. Add the oil in the instant pot and press Sauté.
3. Then add the pureed onion mixture and cook for 2 to 3 minutes.
4. Add the spices and cook for 1 minute.
5. Press Cancel and stir in cauliflower and water.
6. Cover and lock the lid and press Manual.
7. Cook under Low Pressure for 2 to 3 minutes.
8. Press Cancel and carefully do a Quick release.
9. Remove the lid and serve.

Nutritional Facts Per Serving

- Calories: 74
- Fats: 1.7g
- Carb: 3.37g
- Protein: 4.5g

Shrimp and Tomato Casserole

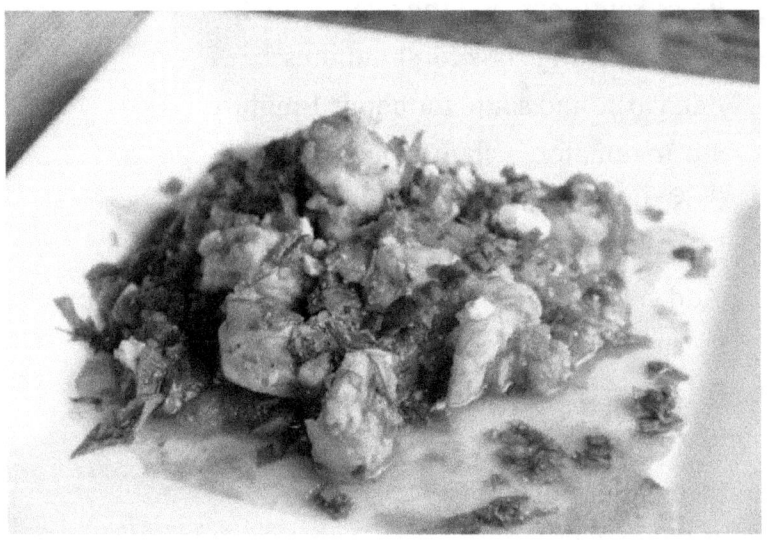

Total time: 30 minutes

Servings: 4

Ingredients

- Shrimp – 1 ½ pound, peeled and deveined
- Tomatoes – 1 ½ pound, chopped
- Olive oil – 2 tbsp.
- Veggie broth – ½ cup
- Chopped cilantro – ¼ cup
- Lime juice – 2 tbsp.
- Jalapeno – 1, diced
- Onion – 1, diced
- Shredded cheddar cheese – 1 cup
- Minced garlic – 1 tsp.

Method

1. Press Sauté, and add the oil into the IP.
2. Add onion and cook for 3 minutes.
3. Add garlic and sauté for about 1 minute.
4. Stir in tomatoes, cilantro, and broth.
5. Close the lid and cook for High for 9 minutes.
6. Do a natural pressure release.
7. Add shrimp and jalapeno. Cook on High for 2 minutes.
8. Release pressure quickly and stir in cheddar.
9. Drizzle with lemon juice and serve.

Nutritional Facts Per Serving

- Calories: 300
- Fat: 16g
- Carb: 8g
- Protein: 22g

Cheesy Spinach

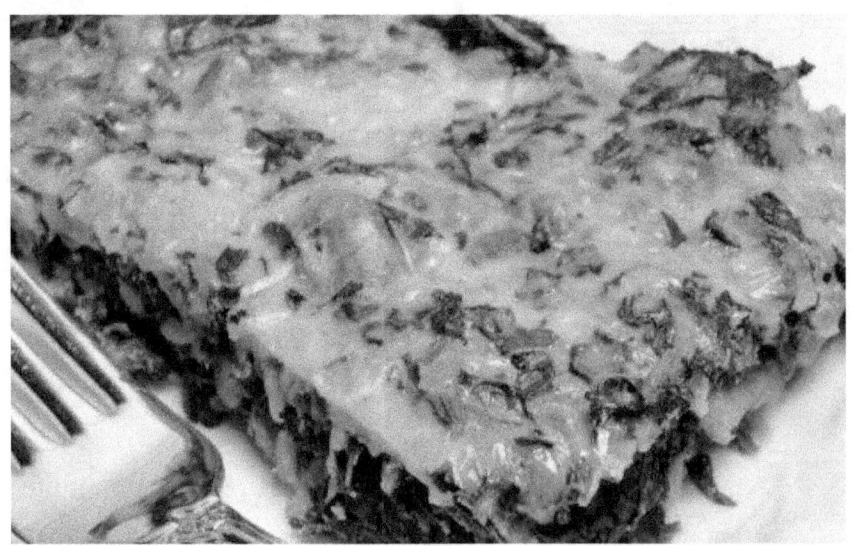

Total time: 25 minutes
Servings: 4

Ingredients
- Spinach – 2 lbs. chopped
- Eggs – 3 large
- Vegetable stock – 1 cup
- Parmesan cheese – ¼ cup, grated
- Chili pepper – 1 small, finely chopped
- Onion powder – 1 tsp.
- Garlic powder – ¼ tsp.
- Chili powder – ¼ tsp.
- Salt – 1 tsp.
- Cayenne pepper – ¼ tsp.

Method

1. Place the spinach in the instant pot. Add the vegetable broth and 1 cup of water. Sprinkle with salt and close the lid.
2. Press Manual, set the timer for 5 minutes, and cook on High pressure.
3. When done, do a quick release and open the pot.
4. Press Sauté and add chili pepper. Sprinkle with cayenne pepper, salt, chili powder, onion powder, and garlic powder.
5. Give it a good stir and cook until half reduces the liquid, about 5 minutes.
6. Poach the eggs on top of the spinach and sprinkle all with Parmesan cheese
7. Turn off the pot and serve.

Nutritional Facts Per Serving

- Calories: 169
- Fats: 8.7g
- Carb: 4.7g
- Protein: 16.8g

Italian Salmon

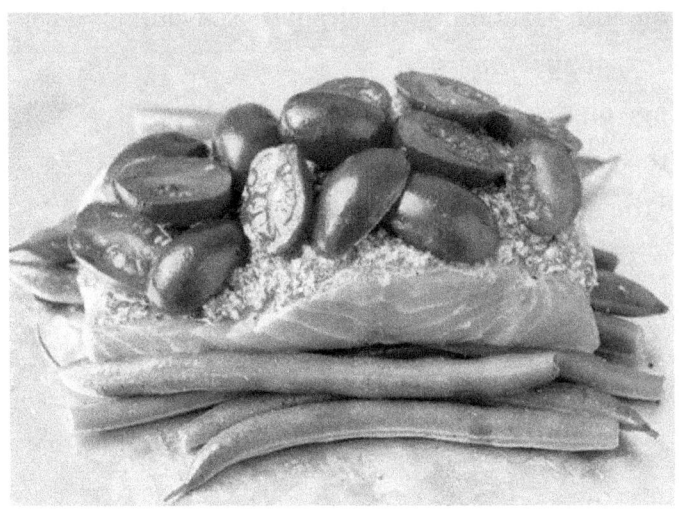

Total time: 10 minutes

Servings: 4

Ingredients

- Salmon fillets – 4 (2 to 3 ounces each)
- Water – 1 cup
- Rosemary sprig – 1
- Olive oil – 2 tbsp.
- Italian seasoning – 1 tsp.
- Pepper – ¼ tsp.
- Salt – ¼ tsp.
- Garlic powder – ¼ tsp.
- Halved cherry tomatoes – 1 cup
- Asparagus spears – 15 ounces

Method

1. Pour the water into the Instant Pot.
2. Season the salmon with Italian seasoning, garlic powder, pepper, and salt.
3. Arrange on the rack.
4. Add the rosemary sprig on top.
5. Place the asparagus spears over.
6. Top with cherry tomatoes.
7. Close the lid and cook on High for 3 minutes.
8. Do a quick release and transfer to a plate.
9. Drizzle with olive oil
10. Serve.

Nutritional Facts Per Serving

- Calories: 470
- Fat: 31g
- Carb: 4.6g
- Protein: 43g

Seafood Paella

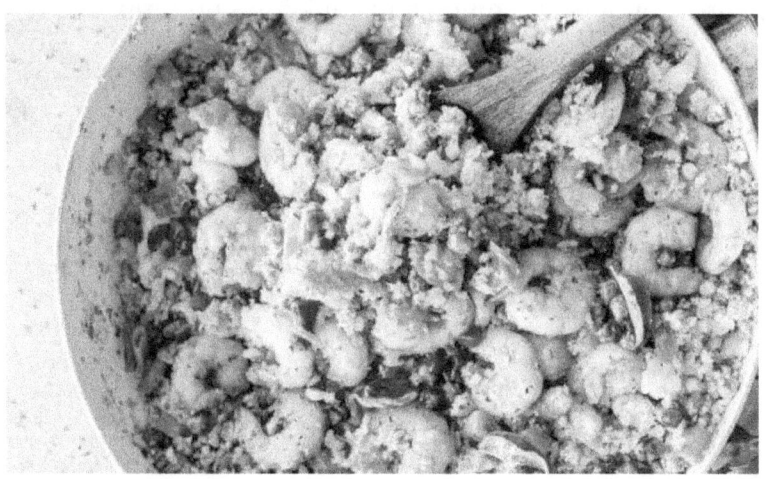

Total time: 30 minutes

Servings: 4

Ingredients

- Chopped fish – 1 cup
- Shellfish – 2 cups (calms, mussels, shrimp)
- Cauliflower rice – 2 cups
- Red bell pepper – 1, diced
- Ghee – 1 tbsp.
- Green bell pepper – 1, diced
- Onion – 1, sliced
- Fish stock – 4 cups
- A pinch of saffron
- Salt and pepper to taste

Method

1. Melt the ghee in the IP.
2. Add peppers and onion and cook for 3 minutes.
3. Stir in the stock, rice, fish, and saffron.
4. Close the lid and cook for 2 minutes on High.
5. Release pressure naturally.
6. Add the shellfish (do not stir) and close the lid.
7. Cook for 3 minutes more.
8. Let the pressure drop naturally.
9. Serve.

Nutritional Facts Per Serving

- Calories: 156
- Fat: 4.5g
- Carb: 5g
- Protein: 15g

Vegetable Stir-Fry

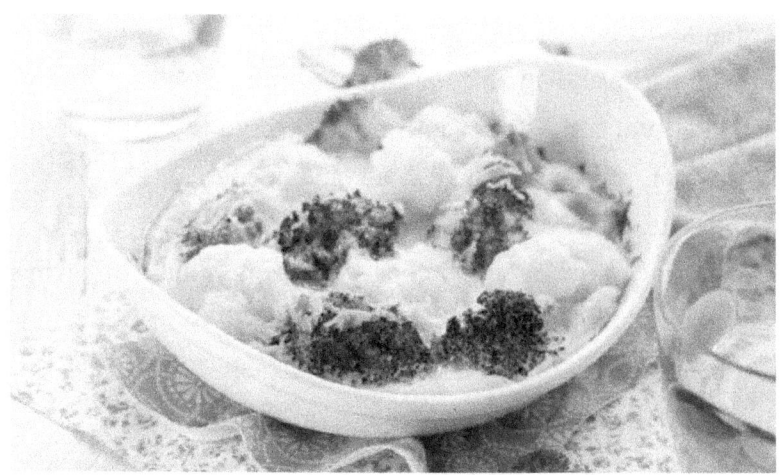

Total time: 20 minutes
Servings: 3

Ingredients
- Cauliflower – 2 cups, chopped
- Broccoli – 1 cup, chopped
- Garlic – 3 cloves, finely chopped
- Olive oil – 1 tbsp.
- Eggs – 2
- Salt – ½ tsp.
- Black pepper – ¼ tsp. ground
- Red pepper flakes – ¼ tsp.
- Onion powder – ¼ tsp.

Method

1. Grease the stainless steel insert with olive oil and press Sauté.
2. Add garlic and stir-fry for 2 minutes.
3. Add broccoli and cauliflower. Sprinkle with onion powder, red pepper flakes, salt, and pepper.
4. Stir and cook for 5 minutes.
5. Add ¼ cup of water and cook for 5 more minutes. Stirring occasionally.
6. Poach the egg on top and season with salt.
7. Cook for 2 to 3 minutes and turn off the pot.
8. Transfer to a serving plate.
9. Serve.

Nutritional Facts Per Serving

- Calories: 115
- Fats: 7.8g
- Carb: 4.3g
- Protein: 6.1g

Sockeye Salmon

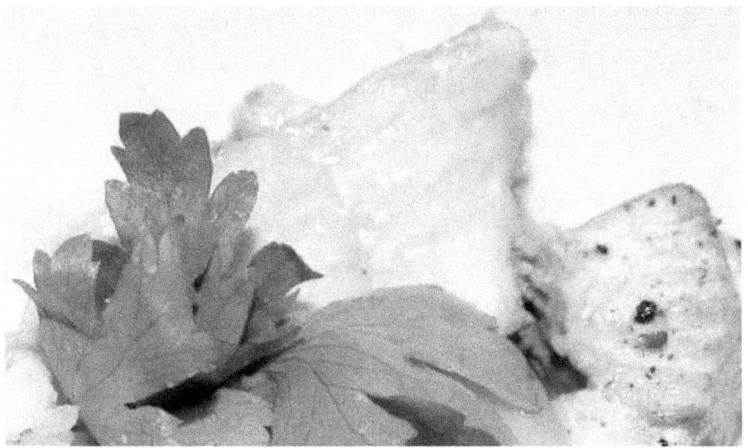

Total time: 10 minutes **Servings:** 4

Ingredients

- Dijon mustard – 1 tsp.
- Garlic powder – 1 tsp.
- Onion powder – ¼ tsp.
- Garlic – 1 clove, minced
- Salmon fillets – 4 (2 to 3 ounce each)
- Lemon juice – 1 tbsp.
- Salt and pepper to taste
- Water – 1 ½ cups

Method

1. Combine the lemon juice, minced garlic, garlic powder, onion powder, and mustard in a small bowl.
2. Brush the mixture over the salmon.

3. Pour the water into the IP and lower the rack.

4. Arrange the salmon on the rack and close the lid.

5. Cook on High for 4 minutes.

6. Do a quick pressure release

7. Serve.

Nutritional Facts Per Serving
- Calories: 195
- Fat: 10g
- Carb: 1g
- Protein: 24g

Haddock and Cheddar

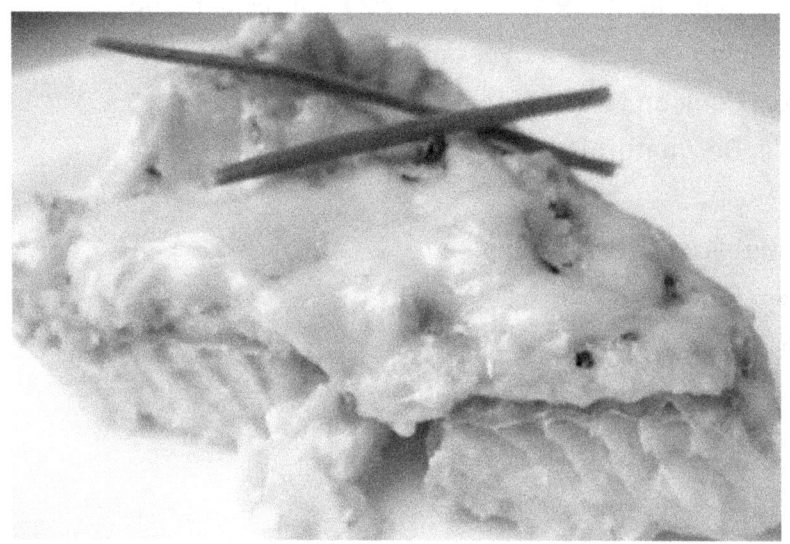

Total time: 30 minutes

Servings: 4

Ingredients

- Haddock fillets – 12 ounces
- Butter – 1 tbsp.
- Heavy cream – ½ cup
- Cheddar cheese – 5 ounces, grated
- Diced onions – 3 tbsp.
- Garlic salt – ¼ tsp.
- Pepper – ¼ tsp.

Method

1. Melt the butter in the IP on Sauté.

2. Sauté the onions for 2 minutes.

3. Season the fish with salt and pepper.

4. Place in the IP and cook for 2 minutes per side.

5. Pour the cream over and top with the cheese.

6. Cook on Manual for 5 minutes.

7. Do a natural pressure release.

Nutritional Facts Per Serving

- Calories: 195
- Fat: 18g
- Carb: 5.5g
- Protein: 18g

Cheesy Broccoli

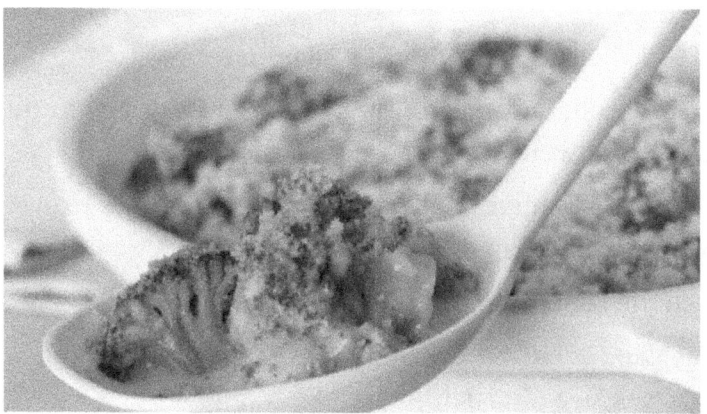

Total time: 25 minutes
Servings: 2

Ingredients

For broccoli

- Broccoli florets – 2 cups
- Olive oil – 1 tbsp.
- Garlic powder – 2 tsp.
- Smoked paprika – ½ tbsp.
- Salt and freshly ground black pepper

Sauce

- Butter – 3 tbsp.
- Almond flour – 2 tbsp.
- Unsweetened almond milk – ½ cups
- Shredded cheddar cheese – 1 cup

- Garlic powder – 1 tsp.
- Salt to taste

Method

1. For broccoli: add all the ingredients into a bowl and toss to coat well.
2. Arrange a steamer basket in the bottom of the instant pot and pour 1 cup of water.
3. Place the broccoli into the steamer basket.
4. Cover and lock the lid and press Manual. Cook under Low Pressure for 10 minutes.
5. Press Cancel and do a Natural release.
6. Meanwhile, for the cheese sauce: in a bowl melt butter over medium heat.
7. Add flour and beat well.
8. Slowly add almond milk and beat continuously.
9. Cook until thickened, about 2 to 3 minutes. Stirring continuously.
10. Add garlic powder, cheese, and salt and stir until smooth.
11. Remove the lid and transfer broccoli on serving plates.
12. Top with cheese sauce and serve.

Nutritional Facts Per Serving

- Calories: 536
- Fats: 47.9g
- Carb: 5g
- Protein: 19.3g

Vegetable Curry

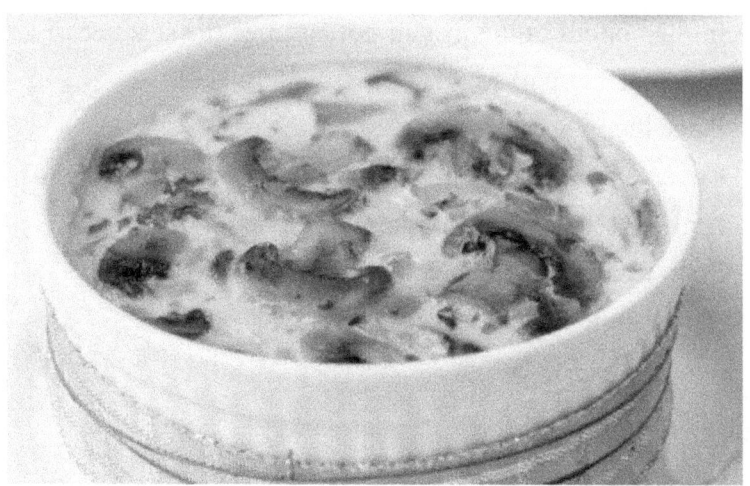

Total time: 42 minutes

Servings: 4

Ingredients
- Sliced fresh mushrooms – 3 cups
- Minced garlic – ½ tsp.
- Salt to taste
- Ground coriander – ¼ tsp.
- Ground cumin – ¼ tsp.
- Ground turmeric – ¼ tsp.
- Red chili powder – ¼ tsp.
- Unsweetened coconut milk – ½ cup
- Plain Greek yogurt – ¼ cup

Method

1. Add all the ingredients in a Pyrex dish and stir to combine.
2. In the bottom of the instant pot, arrange the steamer trivet and pour 1 cup of water.
3. Place the Pyrex dish on top of the trivet.
4. Cover and lock the lid and press Manual. Cook under High Pressure for 27 minutes.
5. Press Cancel and do a Natural release.
6. Remove the lid and serve.

Nutritional Facts Per Serving

- Calories: 93
- Fats: 7.6g
- Carb: 2.22g
- Protein: 3.3g

Dinner

Beef Kale Patties

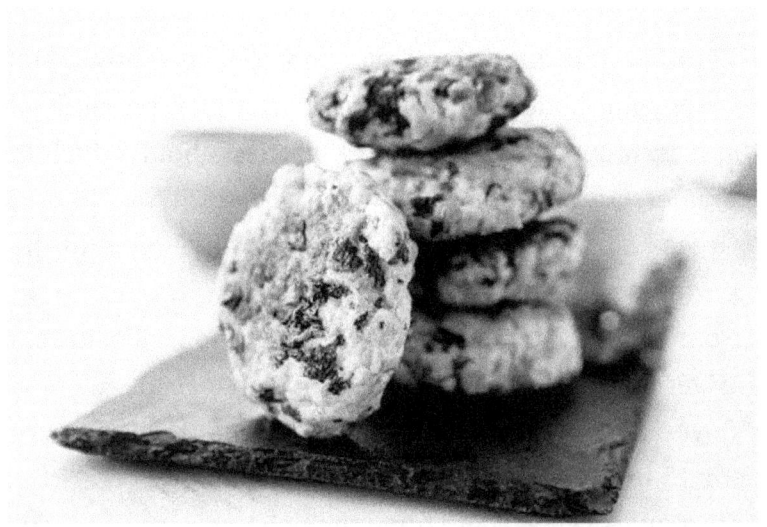

Total time: 25 minutes

Servings: 4

Ingredients

- Ground beef – 1 lb.
- Fresh kale – 1 cup, finely chopped
- Egg – 1, beaten
- Almond flour – 1 tbsp.
- Olive oil – 1 tbsp.

Spices

- Dried rosemary – ½ tsp. ground
- Dried oregano – ½ tsp. ground

- Sea salt – 1 tsp.
- Black pepper – ½ tsp. ground
- Water – 1 cup

Method

1. Combine the flour, egg, kale, and beef in a bowl. Mix with your hand until mixed well. Add flour and all spices. Mix and shape about 8 patties, about 2-inch in diameter.
2. Grease a fitting springform pan with olive oil. Add the patties and set aside.
3. Pour 1-cup water in the inner pot of the IP. Position a trivet on the bottom and place the pan on top.
4. Cover and press Manual and cook on High-pressure for 15 minutes.
5. Do a quick release and open the pot.
6. Cool and serve.
7. Optionally, brown the patties on Sauté mode for 1 minute on both sides.

Nutritional Facts Per Serving

- Calories: 279
- Fat: 12.7g
- Carb: 1.9g
- Protein: 36.9g

Beef Roast

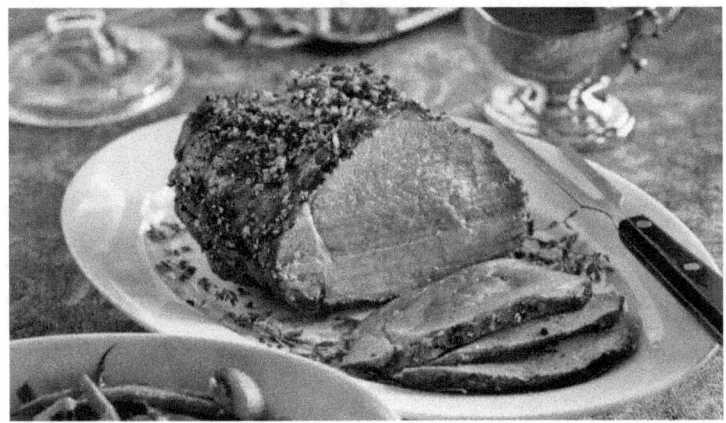

Total time: 1 hour
Servings: 4

Ingredients

- Grated ginger – 1 tsp.
- Beef roast – 2 pounds
- Whole cloves – 4
- Thyme – 1 tsp.
- Garlic powder – 1 tsp.
- Pepper – ¼ tsp.
- Salt – ½ tsp.
- Water – 1 cup

Method

1. Combine all the spices and rub into the meat.
2. Stick the cloves into the beef.
3. Place the beef inside the IP.

4. Pour the water around it.
5. Close the lid and press Manual.
6. Cook on High for 45 minutes.
7. Transfer the beef to a cutting board and shred it with two forks.
8. Serve.

Nutritional Facts Per Serving

- Calories: 710
- Fat:
- Carb: 1.1g
- Protein: 55g

Beef Chuck Roast

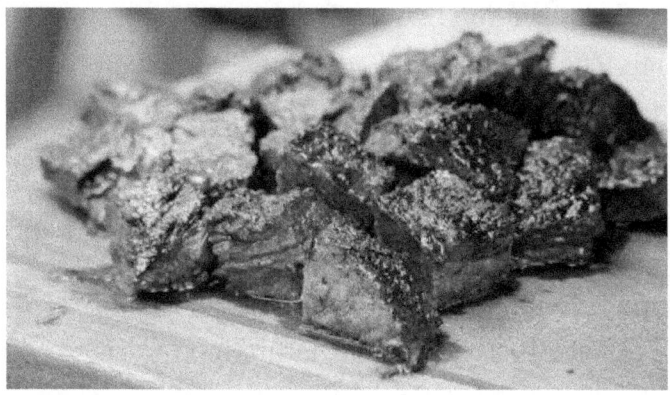

Total time: 45 minutes

Servings: 3

Ingredients

- Beef chuck roast - 1 ½ lb. boneless, cut into bite-sized pieces
- Garlic – 2 cloves, minced
- Butter – ½ tbsp.
- Beef broth – 1 cup
- Tomatoes – ½ cup, diced
- Onion – ½, chopped

Spices

- Black pepper – ½ tsp. ground
- Sea salt to taste
- Fresh oregano – ½ tsp. chopped
- Dried basil – ¼ tsp. ground

Method

1. Melt the butter in the IP over Sauté setting.
2. Add onions and garlic and cook for 3 to 4 minutes or until onions are translucent.
3. Add meat and cook for 5 minutes on each side.
4. Add tomatoes and all the spices. Pour in the broth and cover with the lid.
5. Press manual and cook for 25 minutes on High.
6. Once cooked, release pressure naturally.
7. Open the pot and transfer the meat to a serving plate.
8. Enjoy.

Nutritional Facts Per Serving

- Calories: 651
- Fat: 49.2g
- Carb: 2.2g
- Protein: 46.2g

Duck Breast with Prosciutto

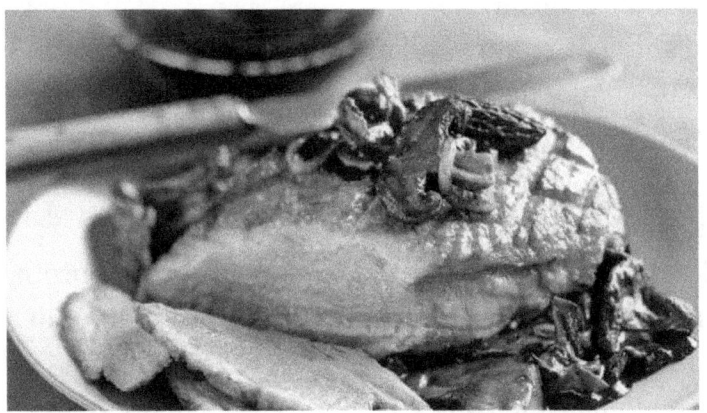

Total time: 50 minutes
Servings: 4

Ingredients

- Duck breasts – 1 lb.
- Shallot – 1, finely chopped
- Garlic cloves – 2, crushed
- Duck fat – ½ cup
- Chicken broth – 4 cups
- Prosciutto – 7 oz. chopped
- Fresh parsley – 2 tbsp. finely chopped
- Apple cider vinegar – 3 tbsp.
- Cremini mushrooms – 1 cup
- Orange zest – 1 tbsp.

Spices

- Sea salt – 1 tsp.
- White pepper – ½ tsp. freshly ground

Method

1. Press Sauté and add the duck fat. Stir constantly and slowly melt the fat.
2. Add the garlic and shallots. Cook and stir for 2 to 3 minutes. Add the mushrooms and continue to cook until the liquid has evaporated.
3. Add the prosciutto and stir well. Briefly brown on all sides and press Cancel.
4. Add the meat into the pot and pour in the broth. Sprinkle with orange zest and spices. Pour in the cider and seal the lid.
5. Press Manual and cook 20 minutes on High pressure.
6. Once cooked release pressure naturally and open the lid.
7. Sprinkle with parsley and cover for 10 minutes before serving.

Nutritional Facts Per Serving

- Calories: 496
- Fat: 34.3g
- Carb: 3.5g
- Protein: 40.9g

Beef Stroganoff

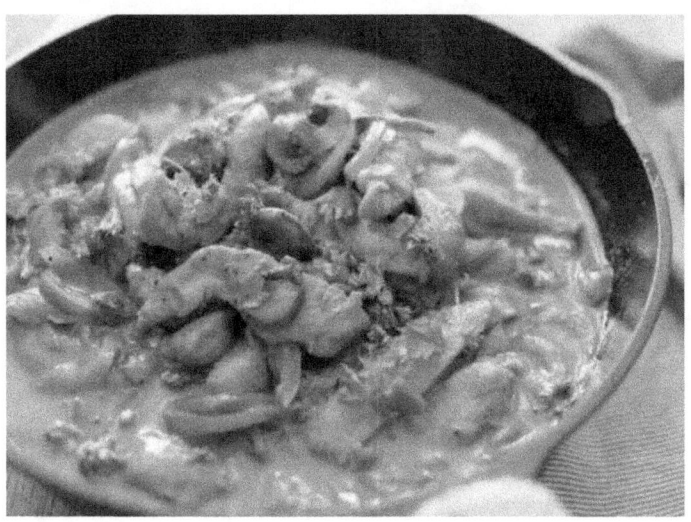

Total time: 20 minutes

Servings: 4

Ingredients

- Small onion – 1, diced

- Garlic – 2 cloves, crushed

- Bacon – 2 rashers, diced

- Beef Sirloin Steak – 1 lb. (cut into ½ inch strips)

- Smoked paprika – 1 tsp.

- Tomato paste – 3 tbsp.

- Beef broth – 1 cup

- Mushrooms – ½ lbs. quartered

- Sour cream – ½ cup

Method

1. Place all ingredients in the instant pot except the sour cream and stir to combine.
2. Place and lock the lid and manually set the cooking time to 20 minutes on high pressure.
3. Naturally release the pressure, and then stir in the sour cream.
4. Serve warm.

Nutritional Facts Per Serving

- Calories: 260
- Fats: 14g
- Carbs: 4.8g
- Protein: 26.5g

Thai Basil Goose Cubes

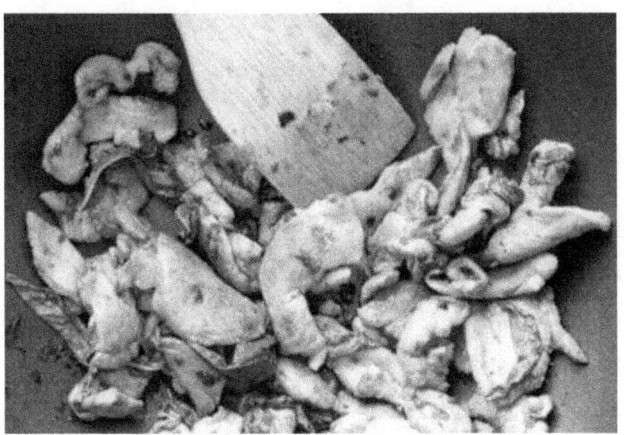

Total time: 40 minutes
Servings: 4

Ingredients

- Chopped basil leaves – ¼ cup

- Cubed goose breasts – 2 cups

- Fish sauce – 2 tbsp.

- Minced chilies – 2 tbsp.

- Minced garlic – 2 tsp.

- Minced ginger – 1 tsp.

- Avocado oil – 2 tbsp.

- Granulated sweetener – 1 tsp.

- Water – 1 ½ cup

- Salt and pepper to taste

Method

1. Heat half of the oil in the IP on Sauté.
2. Add the goose and cook until golden.
3. Transfer to a baking dish.
4. Whisk the remaining oil, fish sauce, chilies, ginger, garlic, and sweetener together.
5. Pour over the goose.
6. Add the basil and season with salt and pepper.
7. Pour the water into the IP and lower the rack.
8. Place the baking dish inside the IP and close the lid.
9. Cook on Manual for 10 minutes.
10. Do a quick pressure release.
11. Serve.

Nutritional Facts Per Serving
- Calories: 192
- Fat: 9g
- Carb: 1g
- Protein: 27g

Salsa Verde Turkey Breast

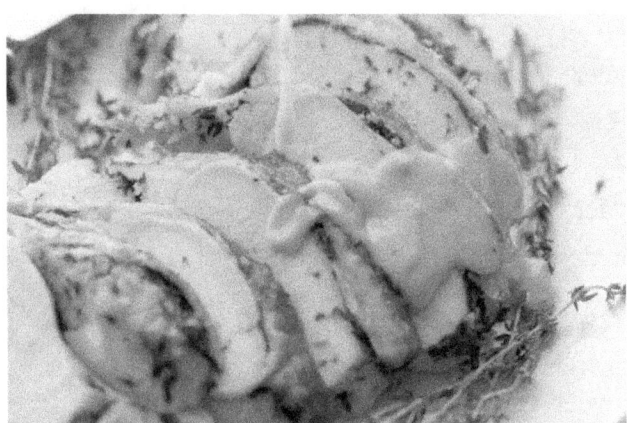

Total time: 35 minutes
Servings: 4

Ingredients

- Medium sized turkey breast – 2, cut in half

- Onion – 1, sliced

- Chicken broth – 3 cups

For the salsa Verde

- Tomatillos – 1 cup, chopped

- Fresh parsley – ¼ cup, finely chopped

- Green chili – 1, finely chopped

- Onion powder – 1 tsp.

- Garlic cloves – 2, crushed

- Olive oil – 3 tbsp.
- Salt – 1 tsp.
- Chili powder – ¼ tsp.

For the rub
- Chili powder – 1 tsp.
- Garlic powder – 2 tsp.
- Onion powder – 1 tsp.
- Salt – 1 tsp.
- Cumin powder – ½ tsp.

Method

1. Combine the garlic powder, chili powder, onion powder, salt and cumin in a bowl. Mix well and set aside.
2. Rinse the meat under cold water and rub well with the spices. Place at the bottom of the IP and pour in the chicken broth. Add the onions and seal the lid.
3. Press Poultry and cook on High for 15 minutes. When cooked, release pressure naturally and open the lid. Remove the meat from the pot and set aside.
4. Remove the broth and press Sauté.
5. Grease the inner pot with olive oil and heat up.
6. Add garlic and green chili. Cook for 2 to 3 minutes and then add the tomatillos along with remaining ingredients for the salsa.
7. Pour in about 3 tbsp. of the broth and simmer for 10 to 12 minutes. Stirring occasionally.

8. Press Cancel and remove the mixture from the pot. Transfer to a food processor and process until smooth.

9. Drizzle over the meat and serve.

Nutritional Facts Per Serving

- Calories: 342
- Fat: 17.7g
- Carb: 5.5g
- Protein: 37.8g

Italian Duck with Spinach

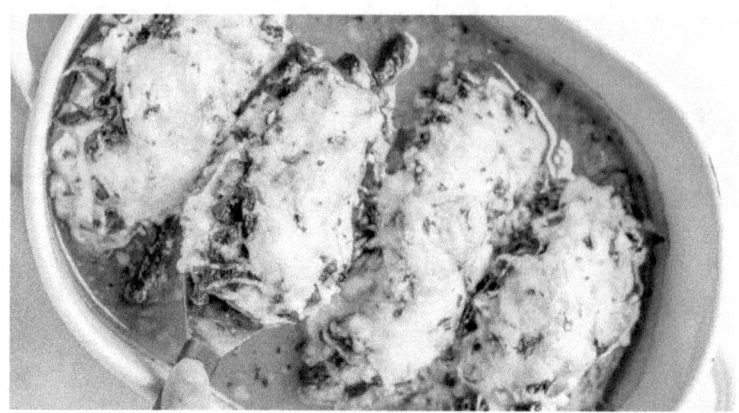

Total time: 40 minutes

Servings: 3

Ingredients

- Duck breasts – 1 pound, halved

- Spinach – ½ cup, chopped

- Chopped Sun-Dried Tomatoes – ¼ cup

- Chicken stock – ½ cup

- Grated Parmesan Cheese – ¼ cup

- Italian seasoning – 1 tsp.

- Heavy cream – 1/3 cup

- Minced garlic – 1 tsp.

- Salt and pepper to taste

- Olive oil – 2 tbsp.

Method

1. Whisk the seasoning, garlic, oil, and salt and pepper together.
2. Rub this mixture into the meat.
3. Place the duck in the IP and cook on Sauté until golden on all sides.
4. Add the stock, close the lid and cook on Manual for 4 minutes.
5. Press Cancel and do a quick release.
6. Stir in the remaining ingredients and cover.
7. Cook on High for 5 minutes more.
8. Release the pressure quickly and serve.

Nutritional Facts Per Serving

- Calories: 455
- Fat: 26g
- Carb: 1g
- Protein: 57g

Turkey with Broccoli

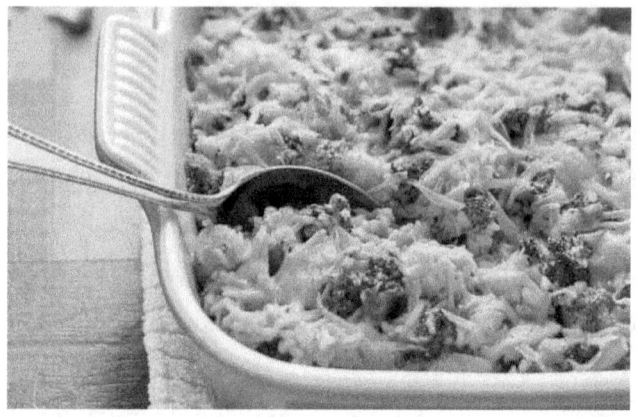

Total time: 50 minutes
Servings: 3

Ingredients

- Ground turkey – 10 oz.

- Broccoli – 1 cup, chopped

- Olive oil – 2 tbsp.

- Spring onion – 1, finely chopped

- Chicken stock – ¼ cup

- Shredded mozzarella – 1 cup

- Sour cream – 3 tbsp.

- Parmesan cheese – ¼ cup, grated

Spices

- Salt – ½ tsp.
- White pepper – ¼ tsp. freshly ground
- Dried thyme – ½ tsp.
- Dried oregano – ¼ tsp.

Method

1. Press the Sauté button and add the olive oil.
2. Now add the spring onions into the hot oil. Cook and stir for 1 minute.
3. Add the broccoli and turkey. Pour in the stock and cook for 12 to 15 minutes. Stirring occasionally.
4. Season with thyme, oregano, salt and pepper and stir in the cheese.
5. Press Cancel and remove from the pot. Transfer the mixture to a baking dish and set aside.
6. Preheat the oven to 350F and bake for 15 to 20 minutes, or until lightly charred.
7. Remove from the oven and chill for a while.
8. Top with sour cream and serve.

Nutritional Facts Per Serving

- Calories: 327
- Fat: 24.5g
- Carb: 1.3g
- Protein: 29.8g

Cajun Beef

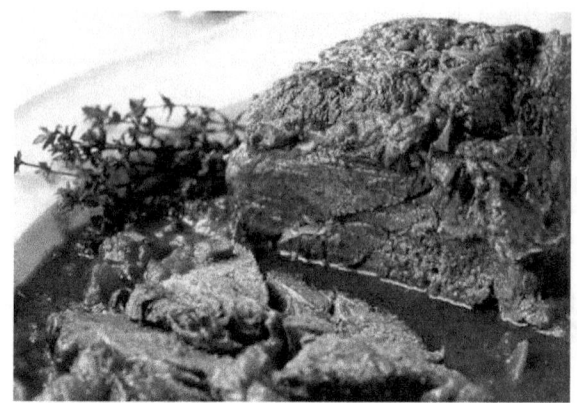

Total time: 20 minutes
Servings: 4

Ingredients

- Cajun seasoning – 1 tbsp.

- Mexican cheese blend – 12 ounces

- Beef broth – 1 cup

- Ground beef – 1 pound

- Tomato paste – 2 tbsp.

- Olive oil – 1 tbsp.

Method

1. Press Sauté and heat the oil.

2. Add beef and cook until browned.
3. Stir in the tomato paste and seasoning.
4. Pour the broth over and close the lid.
5. Cook on High for 7 minutes.
6. Stir in the cheese and cook on High for 5 more minutes.
7. Do a quick pressure release.
8. Serve.

Nutritional Facts Per Serving

- Calories: 400
- Fats: 16g
- Carbs: 4g
- Protein: 33g

Cheesy Chicken with Jalapenos

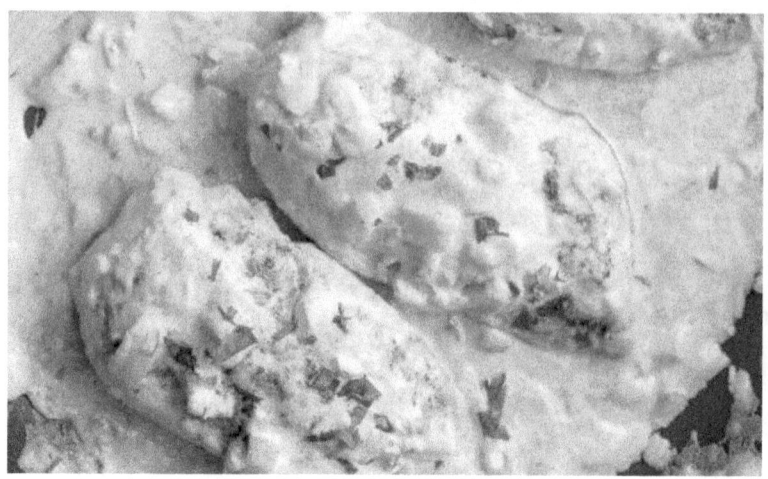

Total time: 20 minutes

Servings: 4

Ingredients

Chicken breasts – 1 pound

Cheddar cheese – 8 ounces, grated

Sour cream – ¾ cup

Jalapenos – 3, seeded and sliced

Water – ½ cup

Cream cheese – 8 ounces

Salt and pepper to taste

Method

1. In the IP, whisk together the water, sour cream, and cheeses.
2. Stir in the jalapenos and place the chicken inside.
3. Season with salt and pepper.
4. Close the lid and cook on Manual for 12 minutes.
5. Do a quick release.
6. Serve.

Nutritional Facts Per Serving

- Calories: 310
- Fat: 26g
- Carb: 4g
- Protein: 20g

Desserts

Nut Flour Cookies

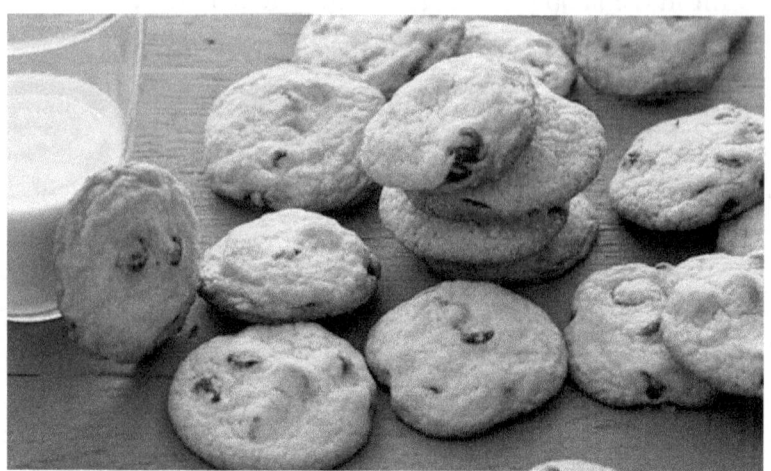

Total time: 40 minutes

Servings: 10

Ingredients

- Almond flour – ½ cup
- Flax meal – ¼ cup
- Coconut flour – ¼ cup
- Almond butter – ½ cup
- Coconut oil – ¼ cup
- Salt – ¼ tsp.
- Swerve – ¼ cup
- Eggs – 3
- Vanilla extract – 1 tsp.
- Unsweetened dark chocolate chips – ¼ cup
- Water – 1 cup

Method

1. Combine coconut flour, almond flour, flax meal, salt and swerve in a bowl.
2. Transfer to a food processor along with coconut oil, almond butter, eggs, and vanilla extract. Process until sandy texture.
3. Transfer the mixture to a lightly floured work surface and fold in chocolate chips. Knead with your hands and shape 10 balls. Press each ball with your hands to form a cookie.
4. Line a baking pan with parchment paper and place cookies.
5. Add 1-cup water in the Instant Pot. Set trivet and place the pan on top.
6. Seal the lid and press Manual. Cook on High for 15 minutes.
7. Do a natural pressure release and open the lid.
8. Transfer cookies to a wire rack and cool.

Nutritional Facts Per Serving
- Calories: 133
- Fat: 11.2g
- Carb: 3.2g
- Protein: 4.2g

Cupcakes

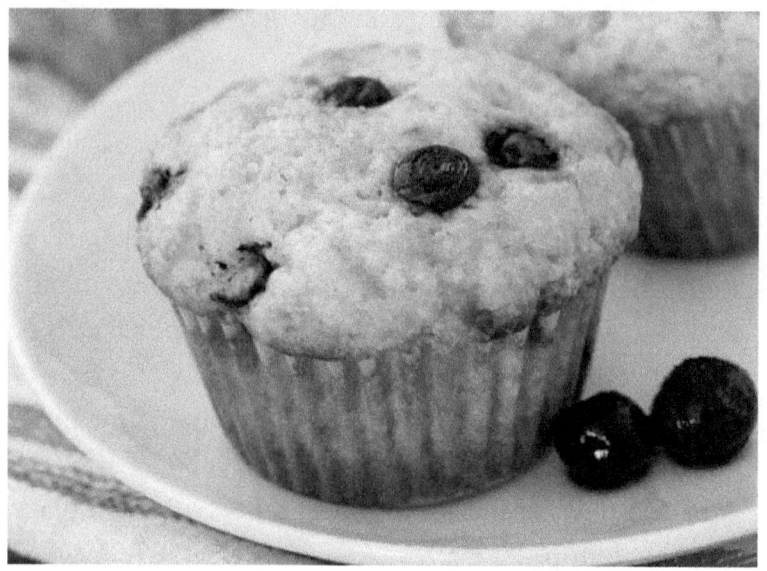

Total time: 35 minutes
Servings: 6

Ingredients
- Almond flour – 2 cups
- Baking powder – 2/3 tsp.
- Baking soda – ¼ tsp.
- Xanthan gum – ½ tsp.
- Swerve – 1 cup
- Eggs – 3
- Almond milk – 1 cup, unsweetened
- Blueberries – ¼ cup
- Butter – 1 tbsp. softened
- Coconut oil – 1 tbsp.

- Lemon zest – 1 tbsp. freshly grated
- Vanilla extract – 1 tsp.

Method

1. Combine all dry ingredients in a large bowl. Mix well and gradually add milk. Beat and add eggs, one at a time. Add coconut oil, butter, lemon zest, and vanilla extract. Mix well.
2. Fold in blueberries and transfer to 12-cup silicone cupcake pan.
3. Add 1-cup water in the instant pot. Set the trivet in the stainless steel insert and place the silicone pan on top. Cover loosely with aluminum foil and seal the lid.
4. Press Manual and set the timer for 25 minutes.
5. When done, do a quick pressure release and open the lid.
6. Remove the muffin pan from the instant pot, and cool completely.
7. Serve.

Nutritional Facts Per Serving
- Calories: 223
- Fats: 20.4g
- Carb: 3.8g
- Protein: 5.9g

Brownies

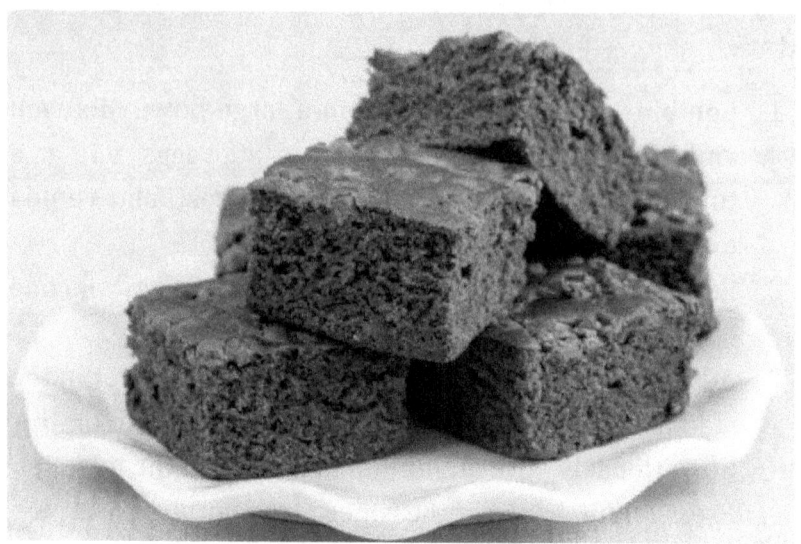

Total time: 30 minutes
Servings: 8

Ingredients
- Cocoa powder – ½ cup, unsweetened
- Unsweetened dark chocolate chunks – ¼ cup
- Cream cheese – 1 cup
- Large eggs – 2
- Coconut oil – 3 tbsp.
- Salt – ½ tsp.
- Swerve – ¾ cup
- Butter – 1 tbsp.

Method

1. In a bowl combine the coconut oil, eggs, and cream cheese. Beat well until smooth. Add dark chocolate chunks, swerve, salt and cocoa powder. Beat until mixed well.

2. Grease a 7-inch cake pan with some oil and line with parchment paper. Dust the paper with some cocoa powder and pour in the butter. Transfer the mixed ingredients. Flatten the surface and loosely cover with aluminum foil.

3. Add 1 cup of water in the instant pot. Set the steam rack at the bottom of the steel insert and place the cake pan on top.

4. Seal the lid and press Manual. Set the timer for 20 minutes.

5. When done, release the pressure naturally for 15 minutes. Open the lid and remove the pan.

6. Cool and serve.

Nutritional Facts Per Serving

- Calories: 180
- Fats: 17.5g
- Carb: 2.4g
- Protein: 4.8g

Almond Flour, Raspberry Pie

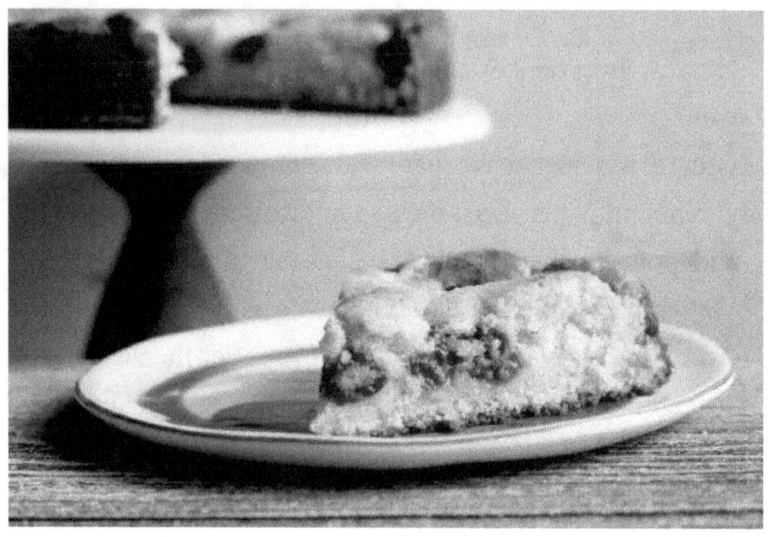

Total time: 40 minutes
Servings: 6

Ingredients

- Almond flour – 2 cups
- Medium peach – 1, sliced
- Raspberries – ¼ cup
- Eggs – 4 large
- Butter – 6 tbsp.
- Baking powder – 2 tsp.
- Salt – ½ tsp.
- Swerve – ¼ tsp.
- Vanilla extract – ¼ tsp.
- Lemon zest – 2 tsp.

Method

1. Brush a 7-inch cake pan with oil and line with parchment paper. Set aside.
2. Whisk the eggs and swerve together in a bowl. Set aside.
3. Combine all the remaining dry ingredients in another bowl and mix well.
4. Slowly pour in the egg mixture, mixing constantly. Then add the remaining ingredients. Transfer to a mixing bowl and beat 2 minutes on medium speed.
5. Pour the mixture into the prepared cake pan and shake a few times to flatten the surface. Wrap with some aluminum foil.
6. Add 1 cup water in the instant pot. Set the trivet at the bottom of the stainless steel insert and place the wrapped pan on top.
7. Seal the lid and press Manual. Set the timer for 25 minutes.
8. Do a quick release when done.
9. Open the lid and remove from pan.
10. Cool and serve.

Nutritional Facts Per Serving

- Calories: 221
- Fats: 19.4g
- Carb: 4.4g
- Protein: 6.6g

Strawberry Cake

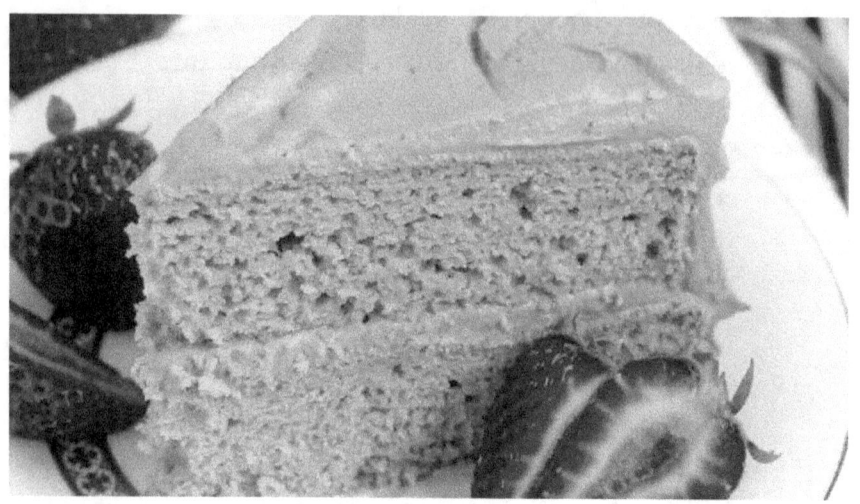

Total time: 35 minutes

Servings: 6

Ingredients

- Almond flour – 2 cups
- Coconut flour – 1 cup
- Unsweetened cocoa powder – ¼ cup
- Baking soda – 1 tsp.
- Baking powder – ½ tsp.
- Salt – ½ tsp.
- Unsweetened almond milk – 1 cup
- Eggs – 3
- Egg whites – 2
- Whipped cream – 3 cups, sugar-free
- Stevia extract – 1 tsp.

- Strawberry extract – 2 tsp.
- Water – 1 cup

Method

1. Line a 7-inch springform pan with parchment paper and set aside.
2. Combine the coconut flour, almond flour, cocoa powder, baking soda, baking powder, and salt in a mixing bowl. Mix well and gradually add milk.
3. Beat on high speed with a hand mixer.
4. Add the eggs one at a time and beat constantly.
5. Finally, add the egg whites and mix well.
6. Transfer the batter to the prepared springform pan and flatten the surface with a spatula. Cover loosely with some aluminum foil.
7. Add 1-cup water in the Instant Pot. Set the trivet in the stainless steel insert and gently place the springform on top.
8. Cover and press Manual, and set timer for 20 minutes.
9. Release the pressure naturally when done and open the lid.
10. Carefully remove the pan. Place on a wire rack and cool.
11. Meanwhile, place stevia, whipped cream, and strawberry extract in a bowl. Beat with a hand mixer to combine well.
12. Pour the mixture over the chilled crust and refrigerate for 1 hour before use.

Nutritional Facts Per Serving

- Calories: 195
- Fat: 16.4g
- Carb: 4.2g
- Protein: 5.7g

Coconut Cake

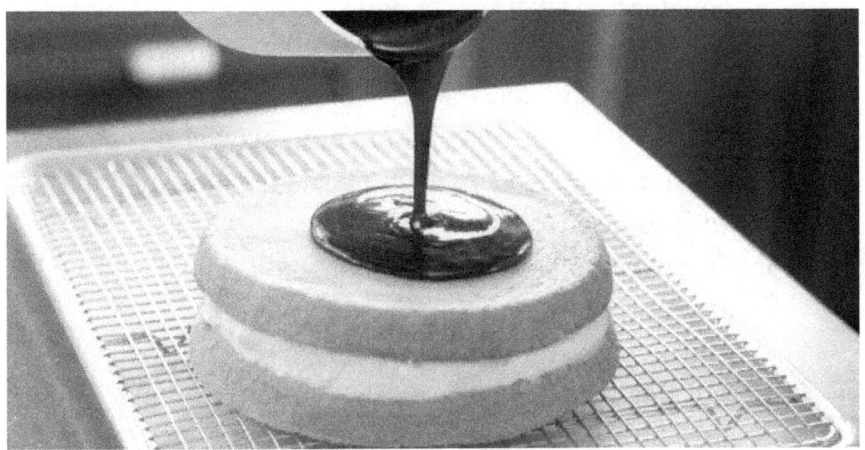

Total time: 50 minutes

Servings: 8

Ingredients

- Coconut flour – 1 cup
- Almond meal – 2/3 cup
- Baking powder – 1 tsp.
- Coconut oil – 1 cup, divided
- Eggs – 2
- Swerve – ¼ cup
- Vanilla extract – 1 tsp.
- Cocoa powder – ¼ cup, unsweetened
- Stevia powder – 1 tsp.
- Whipped cream – 1 cup
- Water – 1 cup

Method

1. Combine the almond meal, coconut flour, baking powder and swerve in a bowl.
2. Add the eggs one by one and beat on medium speed with a hand mixer.
3. Now add 2/3 cup coconut oil and mix well.
4. Brush a 7-inch springform pan with some oil and dust with some cocoa powder.
5. Transfer the batter into the pan and tightly wrap with aluminum foil.
6. Add 1 cup water in the Instant Pot.
7. Set the trivet at the bottom and put the wrapped springform on top.
8. Seal the lid and cook 25 minutes on Manual.
9. Do a quick release when done.
10. Open the lid, remove and cool the cake.
11. Meanwhile, press the Sauté on the Instant Pot.
12. Add the remaining coconut oil, cocoa powder, stevia powder, and vanilla extract.
13. Stir vigorously and add the whipped cream.
14. Cook for 1 minute and remove the chocolate sauce from the Instant Pot.
15. Drizzle the chilled cake with chocolate sauce and refrigerate for 1 hour.
16. Serve.

Nutritional Facts Per Serving
- Calories: 426
- Fat: 39.3g
- Carb: 7.3g
- Protein: 6.6g

Almond Bars

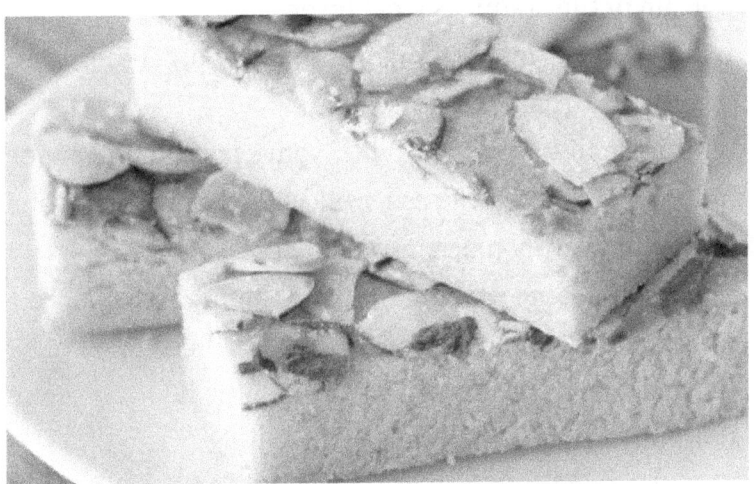

Total time: 20 minutes

Servings: 6 bars

Ingredients

- Almond flour – 1 ¼ cup
- Coconut flour – ¼ cup
- Coconut oil – ½ cup
- Almond butter – 2 tbsp.
- Salt – ¼ tsp.
- Swerve – 3 tbsp.
- Vanilla extract – 1 tsp.
- Eggs – 2
- Water – 1 cup

Method

1. Place the trivet in the IP and add 1-cup water at the bottom of the stainless steel insert.
2. Combine the ingredients in a food processor and process until sandy texture.
3. Line a small baking pan with some parchment paper and add the dough. Press well with the palm of your hands and gently place in your Instant Pot.
4. Cover with some parchment paper and seal the lid.
5. Press Manual and cook for 15 minutes on High.
6. Release pressure naturally and open the lid.
7. Carefully remove and chill.
8. Slice into 6 bars and refrigerate for 1 hour before serving.

Nutritional Facts Per Serving
- Calories: 253
- Fat: 25.7g
- Carb: 1.5g
- Protein: 4.6g

Vanilla Cupcakes with Frosting

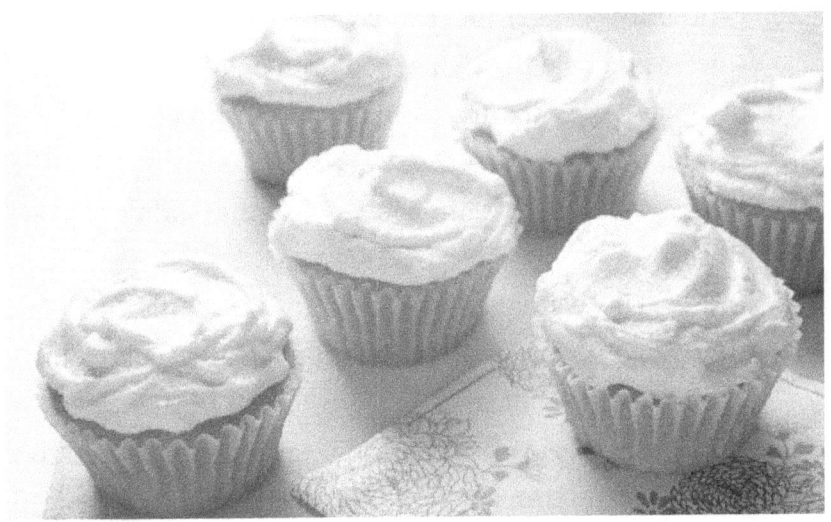

Total time: 30 minutes

Servings: 8

Ingredients

- Butter – ½ cup, softened
- Eggs – 3
- Almond flour – 1 ½ cup
- Swerve – ½ cup
- Vanilla extract – 2 tsp. divided in half
- Baking powder – 1 ½ tsp.
- Cream cheese – 1 cup
- Whipping cream – ¼ cup
- Powdered erythritol - 3 tbsp.

Method

1. Combine almond flour and swerve in a bowl.
2. Add butter, eggs, and 1 tsp. vanilla extract. Use a hand mixer and beat on high speed until mixed.
3. Transfer the mixture to 8 silicon muffin cups and set aside.
4. Place the trivet at the bottom of the stainless steel insert.
5. Add 1 cup water and gently place the muffin cups on top. Cover loosely with aluminum foil and seal the lid.
6. Press Manual and cook for 15 minutes on High.
7. Do a quick release when done and carefully remove the cups and transfer to a wire rack to cool.
8. Meanwhile, combine the remaining ingredients in a bowl. Beat on high speed until light and fluffy.
9. Top each cupcake with this mixture and refrigerate for 30 minutes before serving.

Nutritional Facts Per Serving

- Calories: 262
- Fat: 25.8g
- Carb: 9.4g
- Protein: 5.5g

Conclusion

Thank you for enjoying **Intermittent Fasting for Women.** Hopefully, we have achieved our main goal and provided you with all of the information you could ever hope for on Intermittent Fasting and how it affects the female form. By the end of this guide, readers should have the skills they need to not only get started on their own unique Intermittent Fasting journey but also be able to do so with confidence in both their fasting schedule and themselves.

Some of the skills featured in the guide that we hope reader's find useful include:

- How to choose the right Intermittent Fasting plan to meet specific health goals

- How to plan or alter exercise routines to be most effective throughout a new fasting plan from helping the body adjust in the first few weeks to making changes to their regular fitness routine based on how the body reacts to Intermittent Fasting

- How to stay focused and determined even through the hardest of days of an Intermittent Fasting lifestyle

- How and when are the best ways/times to make changes or alterations to a personalized Intermittent Fasting plan

From here, the next step is to finish gathering your information and get your first Intermittent Fasting plan together! Fasting can be complex, but the more information fasters have, the better the chances for success become for short-term and long-term health goals. There is not any major hurry to get started with Intermittent Fasting as it is meant to be employed as a lifestyle change, or essentially a lifelong practice that can be:

- Developed based on an individual's current health, wellness, dietary and fitness needs

- Adjusted based on health changes over the years

- Put on pause for necessary circumstances like pregnancy for women or any kind of illness that could be enflamed, rather than helped, by Intermittent Fasting

- Even picked back up again without much frustration or concern when the participant is ready to do so

www.ingramcontent.com/pod-product-compliance
Lightning Source LLC
Chambersburg PA
CBHW060858170526

45158CB00001B/398